Community Midwifery

COMMUNITY MIDWIFERY

a practical guide

Mary Cronk RGN RM NCDN ADM

and

Caroline Flint SRN SCM ADM

Illustrations by Helen Chown BA(Hons) Fine Art

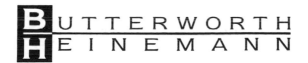

Butterworth-Heinemann Ltd
Halley Court, Jordan Hill, Oxford OX2 8EJ

PART OF REED INTERNATIONAL BOOKS

OXFORD LONDON GUILDFORD BOSTON
MUNICH NEW DELHI SINGAPORE SYDNEY
TOKYO TORONTO WELLINGTON

First published 1989
Reprinted 1989, 1990

British Library Cataloguing in Publication Data
Flint, Caroline
Community midwifery.
1. Midwifery
I. Title   II. Cronk, Mary
610.73'678

ISBN 0 7506 0121 3

Filmset by Eta Services (Typesetters) Ltd, Beccles, Suffolk
Printed and bound in Great Britain by
Biddles Ltd, Guildford and King's Lynn

DEDICATED TO

all midwives – who need to be strong
for the sake of women

Contents

ACKNOWLEDGEMENTS

It is not easy to live with a woman who is writing a book. We would both like to thank our husbands – Joe Cronk and Giles Flint, for their patience, support and cherishing whilst we have been writing it, and our children Mat, Beki, Tom, John and Kate, Peter and Maggie for their encouragement, suggestions and good-natured teasing. Our students past and present have been an inspiration and support to us both and especial thanks go to Rosie Gidlow for her constructive criticism. Nicky Leap made many helpful sugestions and Deb Hughes spent hours on patient sub-editing and making tactful suggestions for improving parts of the original manuscript. Without her invaluable aid and support to both of us, this book would never have been finished.

The women and families we have been privileged to care for during such an intimate time in their lives have, as ever, been a source of wonder, delight and energy to us both and we thank them for their inspiration.

Preface

We have written a practical guide for all midwives working in, or contemplating working in the community – caring for pregnant women in their own homes or in local clinics.

Midwives are already being asked to care for more and more women in their homes. This book will help those who have not done it to any large extent before, and those who have not practised in this way for several years and may need to refresh themselves and revise the skills of caring for women and helping them give birth safely and happily at home.

Midwives currently working in the community may find some fresh ideas for their own practice – and may have some for us. If so we would be grateful to hear from you. We hope the book will also be found useful by midwives working in the community who have been asked to do a home delivery for the first time; students about to go out into the community; midwives working in teams; midwifery managers contemplating setting up teams of midwives to provide continuity of care; and midwives contemplating independent practice.

It is, as the title suggests, a practical guide. It is not a midwifery textbook. We recognise your knowledge of your subject. Our book is about the application of that knowledge in the community setting.

In many areas over the past fifteen years or so, the role of the community midwife has been eroded to that of postnatal nurse, and most maternity care has been concentrated within the walls of maternity units. One consequence of this has been that many midwives who have trained during this period have not developed the confidence to trust themselves to practise safely outside the walls of a hospital. If you are in this situation, you may need to reassure yourself that you do in fact have all the knowledge you need. Consider, then, that during our training we have given care to and supervised 40 pregnant women; palpated 100 pregnant abdomens; performed 50 vaginal examinations; delivered 40 babies after observing 10 normal deliveries; assisted at 40 complicated deliveries, and postnatally examined 100 women and their 100 babies. You **do have** the knowledge and experience. We hope this book will give you the confidence to take your skills into the community.

We also hope that our love for the work we do in the community will spill over into you and that you will find the pleasure we have found in carrying out our professional tasks in the place where pregnancy, postnatal care and possibly the baby's birth really should happen – the home and its locality.

Chapter One

Why Community Midwifery?

Women are often happier and in many cases fare better having their antenatal care in their own homes or somewhere just round the corner. There is now no evidence to support the previously held view that all births should take place in hospital. Indeed, in recent years much research has indicated the advantages of community-based midwifery care. McKee (1982) described how when women received care from locally based midwives and GPs, there was an impressive fall in missed antenatal visits, induction of labour, premature delivery, low birth-weight babies, intra-uterine growth retardation, forceps deliveries, antenatal admission and hospital stays. This care led to a cost-saving to the National Health Service in general, a raising of morale in the women having babies, and a consequent raising of morale in the midwives and GPs as well.

When midwives and obstetricians responded to the Peel Report of 1970, which said that provision should be made for all women to give birth in hospital, we did not just move mothers and their attendant midwives into hospital. We did something else, something much more significant.

Hospitals are places where the sick are cared for by doctors and nurses; care takes place in units called wards. The nursing care is organized and led by ward sisters and delivered by staff and student nurses. Previously maternity patients were largely women with abnormalities of pregnancy (normal pregnancies were managed at home by midwives and GPs). These patients were cared for in wards by obstetricians, midwives and maternity nurses. When we moved the normal pregnant woman into hospital we adopted the existing hospital structure. The woman's care was 'under' an obstetrician and she was 'nursed' on a ward by staff midwives under the management of a ward sister. Her care became fragmented as she progressed from antenatal clinic to the antenatal ward, to the labour ward, to the post-natal ward. The obstetrician who had formerly used his skills to treat abnormal pregnant women now laid down 'policies' for the care of the normal. He usually had a combined obstetrician/gynaecologist consultancy, so was also dealing with the pathology of women, and would come from the ward round on the gynaecology ward to do 'rounds' on the maternity wards.

It is easy to see how the care of women undergoing a physiological process became medicalized when the place of confinement changed. The pregnant woman thought of herself as a 'patient'. The obstetrician thought of himself as the 'doctor in charge', as of course he was on the gynaecological wards. Many midwives with a nursing background found themselves responding as their nurse-training had conditioned them to, and accepting this hierarchical hospital concept of working with 'patients'.

We would like to see this move reversed, but we must ensure that in taking care back into the community setting we do not merely bring the hospital and its attitudes closer to the home. As Newson said in 1985, when writing in *Nursing Mirror*, July 17th 1985, **161**, no. 3; pp. 518–521; about community clinics:

> These clinics are smaller, the waiting times are shorter, and it is to be hoped that GP and midwife will be known to the mother. Low-risk women can, therefore, be transferred from the hospital clinics to community clinics and this will lead to an improvement in care.
>
> Or will it? Does a reduction in travelling and waiting times combined with a known care-giver necessarily lead to an improvement in care? Or is it just possible that the only true improvement is that the women receive inappropriate care more quickly?

The good things we have learnt recently about childbirth need to be retained while we discard many of the 'hospital' attitudes that have dominated care for the past twenty years or so, and look at care as appropriate to the women receiving it.

We care primarily for the woman, her baby and her partner, but community midwifery means more than this. We become involved with the other people who are around when the baby arrives. When a baby is due to be born in a home several things happen within that little neighbourhood – all small things, but things that can contribute to the quality of life of that community. People feel involved; someone will offer the use of a telephone, and having had the phone used will want to know the outcome. Someone will offer to carry the midwife's bags, another will offer to take messages. Neighbours will offer to move their cars, to look after other children, to provide vases for the bunches of flowers arriving. All this is part of the birth and makes us realise how important a part the place of birth plays in life.

As one walks around any big city one sees little plaques on walls: 'John Bloggs was born here', 'Jane Smith was born here'. Many biographies start off with the detail of the subject's place of birth. It is important. Babies being born at home – next door – give life to a community and enable people to develop feelings of neighbourliness which they may not have realised they possessed. Obviously not all babies can be born at home. Not everyone has a home, and not all births are normal. Not every women or her partner wants to have their baby at home. But most couples would appreciate some labour care in their own home, and the support of a midwife they know and trust to accompany them in labour to the hospital.

Some women need the medical and surgical help in pregnancy and labour that only hospital care can provide. These women may be frightened and anxious, so their need to get to know those who will be providing their care is just as great as that of women who are having a normal pregnancy and are able to receive most of their care in familiar surroundings. Women with complicated pregnancies and labours need continuity of care from a small group of midwives who work with and in conjunction with an obstetrician. This arrangement allows the midwives to provide care all the way through pregnancy, labour and the puerperium, and to have the satisfaction of a meaningful relationship with a small number of women who they see throughout their pregnancy and the birth. For most women the relationships forged during this very important time in their lives will never be forgotten. For the doctors, the opportunity to work in unity with a team of committed midwives, who are able to make a relationship with the women they are caring for, will increase their job satisfaction levels and enable them to provide better care.

Klein and his colleagues (1983) showed how advantageous it was for a woman to be visited at home in early labour by a midwife – or even examined in her GP's surgery in early labour when compared with a similar group of women who were given all their labour care in hospital, but not their pregnancy care, which was shared between their GP and community midwife and the hospital. The results showed that women who were assessed in early labour at home spent less time in hospital before they delivered (i.e. they didn't go into hospital until labour was well established), they had less epidural analgesia and fewer forceps deliveries. Their babies had higher Apgar scores and needed less resuscitation, were transferred less often to the special care baby unit, and were more likely to be breast fed for longer.

Another instance of the value of community care by midwives is recorded by Damstra-Wijmenga (1984), who describes what happened to the 1,703 women who lived in Gröningen (north Holland) who had babies in 1981. They were all interviewed about three weeks after their babies were born and she was able to obtain replies from 1,692 of them. The mothers were divided into four categories:

(a) those mothers who had opted for a home confinement;
(b) those who had opted for a hospital confinement followed by a 24-hour stay;
(c) those who had opted for hospital confinement followed by a stay of seven days;

(d) mothers who had to be closely supervised by an obstetrician from the start of pregnancy and had to deliver in hospital owing to an increased risk (primary medical indication).

The fourth group were not studied further. They were the 12% (approx.) who exist in most populations of women who have a primary medical indication for hospital care; they did not have a choice as to where and how they should give birth. The other three groups did have a choice – they were normally healthy women choosing where and how they would give birth.

- 23.4% chose to have their baby at home.
- 32.3% chose to have their baby in hospital followed by a 24-hour stay.
- 32.6% chose to have their baby in hospital followed by a seven-day stay.

There were differences associated with where and how women had chosen to give birth. Even during pregnancy it was noted that women booked for a home confinement were referred less often to an obstetrician during pregnancy (5.6% compared with 10.8% or 12.5%). In women booked for home confinement only 15.6% were referred to an obstetrician during labour compared with 25.3% of women who were booked for hospital delivery.

Of those women referred to an obstetrician during pregnancy only 53.7% gave birth without complications despite the fact that the reasons for their referral would not necessarily require intervention; and interestingly, of the 24 low-risk women who referred themselves to an obstetrician only 54% had uncomplicated births.

It was shown that among those women who had opted for home confinement significantly fewer complications occurred during pregnancy, delivery and puerperium than among those who had their babies in hospital followed by a 24-hour stay there or followed by a seven-day stay in a maternity ward. Morbidity was also lower among the babies

born at home than among those born in hospital. Damstra-
Wijmenga summarises:

> The increasing medicalisation of obstetrics has given rise to the
> notion that it would be 'safer' to deliver in hospital. The safety
> aspect is emphasised in many publications both in the profes-
> sional literature and the lay press. The fact that in a hospital or
> maternity clinic the very surroundings and equipment may give
> rise to iatrogenic complications is apparently overlooked. This
> study has shown clearly that it is a wholly responsible decision
> for a normal healthy woman who is given the right kind of ante-
> natal supervision to have her baby at home, with the least risk of
> complications. It also showed that morbidity was lowest among
> infants born at home.

Shearer (1985) showed the 'added morbidity' associated with
hospital births when he compared the mothers with a similar
group who were booked for delivery at home. More inductions, more episiotomies and second degree tears, and more
Apgar scores of 7 and below were found in the hospital-
booked group.

The booklet produced at the National Perinatal Epidemiology Unit in 1987 by Rona Campbell and Alison Mac-
Farlane, *Where to be Born*, gathers together all the historical
evidence regarding birth at home and concludes that there is
no evidence to support the view that all women should have
their babies in a consultant obstetric unit.

In addition to all this research evidence, there is also an
increasing desire amongst midwives to provide more appropriate care for women in pregnancy and labour, as voiced in
both the Association of Radical Midwives' *The Vision* and
the Royal College of Midwives' *The Role and Education of
the Future Midwife in the UK*. Both these documents advoc-
ate continuity of care associated with midwives working together in small teams (small enough for all the members to be
able to form a meaningful relationship with the women they
are caring for), and care based mainly within the community.
(For more detail see Chapter 15.)

A study in 1987 by Flint and Poulengeris showed the effect

of continuity of care by a small hospital-based team of four midwives, who took responsibility for giving antenatal, delivery and postnatal care to 250 women a year. The results of their study show that, compared with a control group of randomly selected women having normal hospital care, women looked after by midwives who they were able to get to know:

- waited less time in the antenatal clinic.
- felt more satisfied with their antenatal care (which was also less expensive).
- needed less antenatal hospitalisation.
- felt better prepared when they went into labour.
- felt more in control of the situation.
- needed less analgesia.
- had fewer epidurals.
- looked back on their labour much more favourably.
- felt more prepared for motherhood.
- and found being a mother easier.

These results should encourage us to try to provide continuity of care **within hospitals** for those women who cannot be cared for by community-based midwifery practice.

But for the majority of women it seems only reasonable – especially when more and more branches of medicine are providing care in the community, that they should receive care in the comfort and privacy of their own homes, or at a venue which is convenient for them.

References

Campbell, R., MacFarlane, A. (1987). *Where to be Born: The Debate and the Evidence*. Oxford: National Perinatal Epidemiology Unit.

Damstra-Wijmenga, S. M. I. (1984) Home confinement: the positive results in Holland. *Journal of the Royal College of General Practitioners*; 425–31 (August).

Flint, C., Poulengeris, P. (1987). *The Know Your Midwife Report*. London: Heinemann.

Klein, M., Lloyd, I., Redman, C., Bull, M., Turnbull, A. C. (1983). A comparison of low-risk pregnant women booked for delivery in two systems of care: shared care (consultant) and integrated general practice unit. *British Journal of Obstetrics and Gynaecology*; **90**: 118–28 (February).

McKee, I. (1982) Community antenatal care – the way forward. *Scottish Medicine* (April).

Shearer, J. M. L. (1985). Five-year prospective survey of risk of booking for a home birth in Essex. *British Medical Journal*; **290** (23 November).

Chapter Two

Pregnancy Care in the Community

Working with people in their homes and in their neighbour-
hoods can give the midwife a superb opportunity to learn a
great deal about the pregnant women to whom she is offering
care. Many of us coming new to community midwifery after
many years of hospital-based practice are amazed at just how
much easier midwifery is when we know the background, the
family, and the circumstances of our clients.

The first visit to a woman's home is very important. A
successful visit lays the foundation for building that special
relationship between mother and the midwifery service on
which so much depends. We have deliberately said 'the midwifery service', not 'the midwife', because when we visit we
are seen as representing our profession. What we do or say
on that visit can influence that woman's ideas and feelings
about midwives, perhaps for life.

PLANNING THE VISITS

Should the visit be by appointment or 'drop-in'? It is usually
best to make an appointment to visit, tempting though it
sometimes is to save mileage and 'drop in'. Some people are
delighted to have unexpected visitors, but many hate it. So if
you don't know Tracey Smith, your first visit at least should
be by appointment. In some areas you will perhaps have first
met her at an antenatal clinic and can make an appointment
to visit at a mutually convenient time. If the procedure in
your area is that 'bookings' for pregnant women are received
from the hospital, you could telephone her, if she is on the
telephone. Sometimes it is more appropriate to write a letter
introducing yourself and inviting her to phone you to arrange
your visit. Some midwives have a suitable letter or form

printed ready to send out. It is better not to send a postcard as not all pregnancies are known to the family or friends. Likewise, take care when telephoning to ensure that you are speaking to the person concerned and do not divulge who you are or leave messages until the family circumstances are known. It does not need much imagination to see what clangers can be dropped in the course of a well-meaning telephone call!

If the mother is well known to you (perhaps you have been her midwife before) then 'dropping in' may be permissible. Remember, though that a woman with a small child may be extremely busy, and often has her life organized with very little time to spare. When we presume that we can just 'drop in' unannounced and take up an hour of her time we are actually insinuating that her time is not important, and that our time is. We can also be throwing her day into confusion because of the time we have taken up.

THE VISIT

Having made the appointment, we knock on the door. It is very good for us to do this. We don't know what lies behind that door and our feelings must be somewhat similar to the woman entering an antenatal clinic for the first time: a bit unsure of the reception, hoping you will like the people, hoping they will like you, wondering what they will be like.

Fortunately, midwives are usually very welcome visitors in homes. It is our responsibility to maintain that welcome. When we visit a woman to take her history on her own ground it is usually a relaxed and friendly occasion which women have anticipated eagerly. Coffee or tea is usually offered and we start to get to know each other.

Of course you want to know the answers to all the usual questions about the woman's reproductive history, medical history, last period, menstrual cycle. The woman will want confirmation of her expected date of delivery. But don't rush into all this. As you sit there sipping your tea, it is helpful to tell the woman something about yourself, where you live, whether you have any nephews and nieces or children of your own. Tell her your names and ask what she would like to call you, and what she would like to be called. If the woman says that she would like to call you 'Sister Cronk' or 'Mrs Flint' but would like to be called 'Mandy', she is telling us about how she sees our relationship, and how she needs help to develop her self-esteem and a realisation that it is *her* contribution to her pregnancy that is much more important than ours. She needs to see us as a friendly partner in her care, with skills and expertise to offer; an experienced adviser and supporter, not an authoritarian 'expert'.

This woman is going to become someone's mother. She is going to become responsible, either singly or with her baby's father, for bringing up a child to adulthood. She needs to be loving, caring, strong, confident, knowledgeable; to see her child through feeding, teething, walking, talking, potting, playing, cuts and grazes, schooling, growing, and into independence. For some women pregnant for the first time, this first meeting with a midwife can be the start of the process of growing from someone's child into someone's mother.

Having established what we are going to call each other – and we should accept whatever she feels she wants – the visit proceeds. Sometimes one can take it fairly quickly, sometimes there is a need to let the visit take some time. Some women regard this visit as one of inspection and want to show us over the house or flat, and expect us to investigate the state of the lavatory. While one might not altogether relish the role of sanitary inspector it is probably important to go along with this. One woman was overheard to comment on her midwife's first visit that she had spent days preparing for it – and 'she couldn't even be bothered to go upstairs'.

When visiting a woman pregnant for the first time, we can get a general feeling about her attitude to her pregnancy, her fears, her expectations, her needs. Asking both parents how and where they were born and how their siblings were born can give us an indication of what they could be hoping for, or are fearful about, or are dreading.

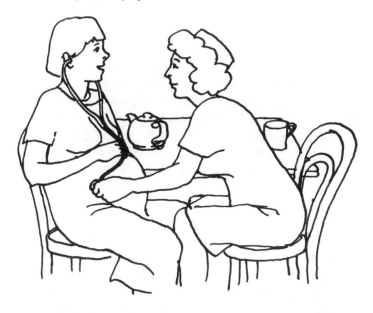

We ask about diet. A useful method of helping a woman identify for herself if she is eating well is to ask, what did she have for breakfast today? lunch? what's for supper? We can then discuss her needs and those of the baby. A woman's financial status will have a great effect on her diet. If she is dependent on income support it will be extremely difficult for her to feed herself adequately. It is very easy for us to prattle on about the value of wholemeal bread, fresh fruit, vegetables, a good source of protein and the importance of good nutrition. We can even write in our notes 'Dietary advice given', but unless we can help a woman work out how to feed herself on the income she has we are failing her. There is some evidence that the present levels of income support do not permit a diet suitable for pregnancy. Perhaps this is something that midwives should be bringing to the notice of the authorities responsible for setting income support levels.

Many midwives will be concerned by women who have strong views about diet. For example, vegans who eat no animal or dairy products whatsoever, or people who eat only certain grains. If the midwife is herself someone without any dietary restrictions it is sometimes difficult for her to understand the views of others and she may be concerned that the woman's diet might lack important nutrients. Most women who adhere to restricted diets have a very good knowledge of nutrition and are only too happy to explain the principles behind what they are doing. Often they have books on the subject that they will lend. It is, nonetheless, important to establish that the diet is not seriously deficient in any important minerals or vitamins. Further reading on this subject can be obtained from The Vegetarian Society. A particularly helpful book is *Rose Elliot's Vegetarian Mother and Baby Book*.

We ask the woman does she smoke? Does her partner? How does she feel about it? We can express our concern for her baby if she or her partner is a smoker, but a first visit is not the time to launch into an anti-smoking tirade. We can show that we understand how difficult it could be to stop, but that there will be lots of help and support available should the couple decide to give up.

We should enquire concerning alcohol intake and give advice based on the latest research.

It can sometimes be helpful to mention that sexual intercourse is perfectly safe throughout normal pregnancies but that sometimes one or other, or both, partners may have a loss of libido. This needs understanding and consideration for each other, and perhaps it could be thought of as a preparation for parenthood, when caring, understanding and consideration for each other are an important contribution to successful parenting.

It is sometimes difficult to know just how much to try to get through in a first visit. A possible check list could be:

- Make friends.
- Identify needs – emotional, financial, social, physical.
- Discuss future programme for antenatal care, where, by whom.
- Discuss place of birth, inform her of the options available.

- Inform the woman of her rights and our responsibilities to her.
- Assess suitability and acceptability of programme offered.
- Ensure that she has all the information she needs at this stage regarding maternity benefits, welfare benefits etc., and that she can read and understand any pamphlets you intend to leave with her.
- Make arrangements for next meeting, and suggest what could be discussed then.
- Mention in an unfrightening way the deviations from normal that a woman should notify her midwife or doctor about immediately. This would include: any vaginal bleeding; itchy, painful, or smelly vaginal discharge; urinary disorders (dysuria, urgency or retention); any abdominal pain.
- Enquire what books, if any, she has read or is reading about pregnancy. It is not unknown for a woman to have got hold of some very out-of-date texts from her mother or an older relative, which may give quite incorrect advice about such things as breast preparation. It is part of our job to be aware of what is available and to advise on a publication suitable for the mother we are speaking to. Some midwives operate a personal lending library.
- Ensure that she has a list of all the antenatal classes being held in the neighbourhood, and encourage her to attend. We can often suggest linking up with others known to us to share transport.
- Remember to make sure that she has had the opportunity to ask questions. Sometimes we are so anxious to make sure that we do not miss out anything important that we forget to say something like 'Is there anything else that you want to ask me?' or 'Are you worried about anything?'

SUBSEQUENT VISITS

As the pregnancy continues the woman and her midwife should form a closer relationship. It is very easy for us to become possessive about 'our' mothers, but it is important that the mother has the opportunity to meet the other mid-wives in the team who will be involved in her care and to develop confidence in all her carers. While visits to the home are vital, some of the antenatal care can be given on the midwives' territory: at a clinic, perhaps shared with the general practitioner, perhaps a clinic run by a team of midwives or shared with a consultant obstetrician, or in our own consulting room.

It is our duty as midwives to ensure that the pregnant woman has all the information available to enable her to make an informed decision about the place of birth and it is our duty to counsel her on the appropriateness of her choice. Chapter 4 describes in greater detail the preparations needed for a woman who plans a home birth.

The woman who plans a hospital birth should have a choice about how long she wants to spend in hospital following the birth. She may ask what the community midwife recommends. In helping the woman make a booking, even a provisional one, we can suggest several things that the woman can consider.

What sort of person is she? Does she enjoy being with other people? Does she like having lots of different people to consult and help her? Will she find it easy sleeping in a room with however many people are in the postnatal wards of the local maternity unit? Will having other new mothers around be of help to her? If she is new to the district perhaps a stay in the postnatal ward will enable her to make friends with people. If she is a first-time Mum will she feel much more secure getting to know her baby in an institutional setting together with other mothers? What are her facilities like at home if she comes home very early? Is there anyone available to help with the domestic chores? The local authority is obliged to provide a home help for newly delivered mothers, either free of charge or at cost price. You should have the telephone number of the organiser of this service in her area.

Many new mothers and babies benefit from coming home early, but for others the time spent in hospital can be a very special private time when they have just got each other, without any other relatives, friends or even other children to intrude except at visiting time. 'Just me and my baby. It will be the only time we have just us two. I can play dollies with him here with no one else around,' a young mother said recently, following the birth of her second child. Even though she was in the middle of a large busy postnatal ward she felt that there she could have a little oasis of time with her new baby before going home to share him with the rest of the family. She enjoyed the communal living of the ward, but was still able to do her own thing with her baby.

Other mothers will feel quite differently; they may be essentially very 'private' people and hate living and sharing living space with others. In the hospital, they can't sleep because of the hustle and bustle at night, and all the other people around them. They can't wait to get home, back to their own bed tucked up beside their baby's father. They want to get to know their baby their way without other mothers and babies around. They find having several different members of staff on different shifts upsetting and confusing. They want the father and other children involved with the new baby right from the start, and find that the visiting hours in hospital, even the most flexible, restrict the family getting together. Most midwives will have seen women who have been persuaded to stay in for a 'rest' but that is the last thing they are having. They can't settle, can't sleep, they don't like the food, they cry, their babies cry, their husbands hover outside sister's office at visiting hours, wondering what's wrong. For this woman going home as soon as possible, with her own known midwife visiting daily and available to consult by phone, can be the right arrangement.

When discussing the length of stay in hospital after the birth it is essential that we should be flexible, and so should our colleagues within the hospital walls. The woman who was 'definitely' coming home four hours after delivery sometimes decides to stay for four days, and the woman who wanted to stay 'at least a week' can decide to leave six hours after the delivery.

Women also need to know that should a longer stay than

had been planned become advisable on medical grounds, for example after a difficult operative delivery, there will be no problem in arranging this.

We may have had the opportunity to meet the husband/partner and other members of the family on our first visit and to have involved them in all that we have done and said. If this has not been possible we should try to meet them soon and involve them in our care. The community midwife should be prepared to work flexi-hours in order to make herself available at evenings and weekends or at times to suit shift workers. If it is not convenient to meet the baby's father for some time, it is often appreciated if we say he should feel free to phone if there is anything that he would like to discuss.

When we ask the woman what her husband's occupation is we are not just attempting to identify her social class for the benefit of the Office of Population Census Studies. We should be looking out for the occupations that could have an effect on the pregnancy. This would include men whose jobs take them away from home for long spells: for example, long-distance lorry drivers, members of the armed forces, airline employees, oil rig workers. The woman whose husband is away for long spells may need extra support, particularly if there are no other family members around. There are certain occupations that carry an increase in stress for wives and girl-friends. We would include prison officers, prisoners, policemen, firemen, junior hospital medical staff. Each community midwife will get to know her patch, its environmental factors and problems.

The woman's own occupation can also have a high stress level: for example, being involved in high finance and having to fly all over the world, working in a canteen or a laundry, or being a nurse and having heavy lifting to do. Unfortunately not all health authorities have occupational health provision for their own staff and it is important to remind the pregnant nurse or doctor or hospital domestic worker that she should be avoiding exposure to anaesthetic gases. It is sometimes helpful for the midwife to liaise with the occupational health service of an employer of a pregnant woman.

We have both learnt the hard way that it is not a good idea to presume relationships when visiting homes. The assumption that the elderly gentleman by the fireside with the toddler on his lap must be grandad ... It took quite some time to restore a relationship with that father! Both of us have had embarrassing moments when we have met a woman and presumed that she was the prospective grandmother only to discover that she was the pregnant mother.

The needs of women and families belonging to minority ethnic groups may sometimes be complex, but as with all the pregnant women you are seeing, the way to find out the woman's needs and expectations is to ask her, and to be open when listening. It can be very problematic when you don't share a language. Much communication can take place through body language, and obviously, it is easier for the woman when she is able to get to know you. At least there is a reassuringly familiar face. But it would be such a blessing if we were all able to communicate with a type of sign language that transcended spoken language.

Throughout the pregnancy we will be seeing the woman at increasingly frequent intervals. The accepted pattern for many years has been:

- From booking to 28 weeks, monthly visits
- 28–36 weeks fortnightly visits
- 36 weeks till delivery weekly visits

We have attempted to discover when this was first set down on the tablets of stone which it certainly seems to be inscribed at the time of writing. Apart from the work of Hall (*Antenatal Care Assessed*, Aberdeen University Press, 1985), we have found little evidence that this regime of care has been submitted to any scientifically based evaluation. It has long been accepted as a 'good thing' and until such time as more research establishes just how good it is we can use it as a guide to good practice, adapting it as necessary to meet the needs of individual women.

DIFFICULTIES

Sometimes we will visit a house that is absolutely filthy. We don't just mean one that we have visited on a bad day. We mean a habitation that is smelly, where there is excreta, decaying food, heaps of mouldering clothes, where the floor covering is unidentifiable but one's shoes stick to it.

Such homes are to be found in cities, in towns, in villages and in rural isolation; and in all social classes, though they are mainly associated with social deprivation and poverty. They can be thought of as 'wear-your-waterproof-underskirt houses'. A wise midwife with whom one of us trained many years ago, referred to such establishments in this way, to stress the importance of going into that home and sitting down. If what one sat down on was likely to be damp and unspeakably horrible, well, one wore a waterproof underskirt and got on with it! It is important to try to identify any cause of the conditions and to enlist other agencies who can help. If there are under-school-age children the family will already be known to the health visitor and it will be important to liaise with her. Sometimes such conditions are a symptom of depression and despair and the case should be discussed with the woman's general practitioner. Sometimes the conditions are associated with alcohol or drug abuse and the midwife should try to identify if there are any problems in these areas. The health visitor may enlist the assistance of the social services department. If the conditions are a health hazard some social services departments provide 'home-makers' who give help, encouragement, and supervision to such households, or 'dirty squads', who will give the house a blitz clean. Perhaps the most difficult thing for the community midwife to accept is that sometimes whatever she does will be ineffective and that any improvement will not last. Our job in these circumstances is to do the best we can within the limits the woman will allow us, and to accept that we will probably not be able to change very much. This woman and her baby are at risk. It is our intervention as midwives that can minimise that risk. This woman needs us as much as any of our cases, probably more than most.

It is important to set goals that are realistic and that have some chance of being reached. We may identify that the food preparation areas are a real health hazard and that the baby's needs for clean nourishment will be best met by breastfeeding. We can put a great deal of energy into persuading her to breastfeed, but we must realistically assess our chances of success and weigh up the factors that we know will predispose to artificial feeding: her family attitudes, the feeding method chosen for other babies, what her friends do. If it is apparent that our chances of persuading her to breastfeed are remote, we might do better for the baby by putting our energy into teaching about the importance of hygiene, in even just a little area in the kitchen that will be used for baby food preparation.

The problem may be that events have overwhelmed a family which cannot cope. A common scenario can be: money is short so the electricity bill isn't paid and the Electricity Board threatens to disconnect the family. They don't read the notice properly, do not understand that they can get help, and the supply is disconnected. Consequently the vacuum cleaner cannot be used, so the place gets dirtier and dirtier. Candles are used, increasing the general grime. The hot water system fails so clothes get soaked and forgotten, and they get dirtier. They all smoke so it gets dirtier. What small amount of energy there may have been initially gets less, and it gets dirtier ... and so the downward spiral goes on. Often such families are ostracised by neighbours, and there may be a history of petty crime. If we do manage to make a relationship with this woman we must guard it carefully and take one step at a time. It is vital to have frequent contact with the other agencies involved and to discuss the case with one's supervisor of midwives.

Most midwives will have encountered women who, for whatever reason, resent being visited, are antagonistic, sometimes even aggressive towards us. It is so easy to be resentful back. Here we are offering to give this woman all our help, our friendship, our expertise, and we are met with suspicion, dislike, and overt rudeness.

Almost invariably the woman who displays this behaviour is afraid: afraid of us taking her over; afraid, because of conditioning by her mother or her sister or a friend, that we will want to do things to her that she will not want us to do. It may be that a previous experience of childbirth has been bad, and she feels she has been badly treated by professionals.

It can take all our communication skills to overcome this attitude. We smile, we are conciliatory. Sometimes it helps to be quite direct and say something like, 'You are obviously upset by my visit. Is it something I have done or not done that has upset you? Please tell me. Would you like me to come back another day?' Sometimes it is a total rejection by the woman of anyone she sees as an 'authority' figure. Maybe this is based on previous experiences, or she may be very young and still going through an adolescent rebellion. Sometimes it is useful to say something like 'You are entitled to my help and it is my job to do everything I can to assist you.' By saying this, you can show that you are offering a service, not coming as a dictator. This is a situation where midwives working together, and meeting regularly in a group to support each other (as we discuss in Chapter 13) have such an advantage. If a midwife is getting nowhere with a family who totally reject her, perhaps a colleague can see the problem more objectively and suggest something she has failed to spot. Or perhaps a different person may succeed in making contact. Sometimes it is our uniforms that are the barrier to communication. It is well worth trying a visit in one's usual clothes.

The whole question of uniform-wearing is a vexed subject. For whose benefit do we wear our blue and grey? We are both of the opinion that uniforms for midwives have little or no place. Yes, we both feel some pride in our uniforms. Yes, we both remember when we first qualified and changed from our pupils' navy to our cornflower blue SCM dresses. But did it really do anything for the people we were giving care to? We know all the arguments about making us recognisable in

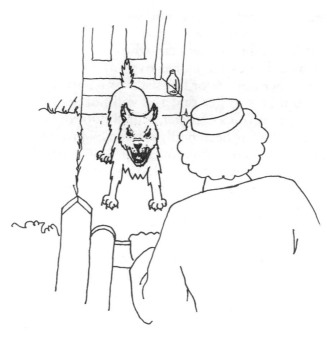

the community, about giving us status (what status?). We can learn from our health visitor colleagues, who say that discarding their uniforms has increased their view of themselves as professional women and has enhanced their relationship with their clients. The only thing to be said in favour of uniform-wearing is that returning to a badly parked car in uniform just might influence the stern traffic warden! We hope that the midwife of the future will not wear a uniform but will dress appropriately for the work she is undertaking, and that she will be in receipt of a salary that will enable her to dress herself for work without having a uniform provided as part of her remuneration.

DOGS, CATS AND OTHER ANIMALS

Some midwives have real anxieties about visiting a home which includes large or small dogs of fearsome aspect. If you know that you are terrified of dogs it is a good idea to mention it if possible when you make your initial appointment to visit, but sometimes we will find ourselves confronted at a garden gate by a vocal toothy canine . . . What to do? Well, if he is making all that noise he is acting as a doorbell and the woman will soon appear to rescue you. If she doesn't and you can't get to the door, she probably isn't at home and you can retreat to your car and telephone or write to make another appointment, at the same time mentioning your encounter with Fido and asking that he be confined when you next visit.

When visiting an animal lover's home the midwife should make an opportunity to give advice about the safeguards that can be taken.

Toxoplasmosis is a disease of cats that very infrequently can infect the human. There is no effective feline vaccine against it. It is spread by the excreta of the animal so the precaution of normal good standards of hygiene and careful disposal of the cat litter tray, if one is used, should be discussed. If there is a dog we should be reminding the family to ensure that the vaccinations are up to date. Most dog diseases do not affect humans but leptospirosis does and it is covered by the standard regular vaccinations.

It is very important that both cats and dogs are regularly dewormed. Round worms are exceedingly common and are present in all puppies at birth. Remind the owners that regular three-monthly deworming of adult dogs, and two-weekly deworming of puppies until they are sixteen weeks old will ensure both the health of their pets, and protect the new baby and any other children. Regular treatment with a good animal insecticide will protect against fleas, lice, and the animal mites that can produce allergic conditions.

Midwives working in rural areas will remind pregnant women to avoid contact with sheep, particularly pregnant ewes and newborn lambs. Their contribution to the work in the lambing sheds should be confined to brewing the tea. It should also be stressed tactfully that their partners should wash thoroughly after tending the sheep and they should be encouraged to put their own contaminated clothing in the washing machine. If the woman *must* handle contaminated clothing she should be advised to wear gloves. Most country-women are aware of these dangers, but newcomers may lack knowledge of the hazards of contacting infection from *Chlamydia psittaci* and other enzootic organisms that have been implicated in spontaneous abortion, renal failure, and blood disorders. The Ministry of Agriculture produce guidelines on the subject and update the information regularly.

THE PREGNANCY PROGRESSES

As the pregnancy progresses we continue our antenatal care monitoring that all is progressing normally, the baby is growing, the woman is remaining in good health. We will see the woman in a variety of settings, her home, at a clinic shared with her general practitioner, in our own consulting rooms or clinic or at a midwives' clinic held at the hospital. We build on what we have learnt already and work on areas of need that we have identified. We consider it essential to good care for the woman to hold her own notes and to have everything that is put into her notes shared with her and understood by her. If we have identified that Sharon Brown smokes 30 cigarettes per day we can record our concern and our advice. Sharon Brown can record her feelings about this and hopefully also her plans to help her baby by either curtailing her smoking or stopping. We would like to see a large column on every antenatal page of every set of notes headed 'Mother's remarks' or 'Mother's views', which the mother could fill in either during or prior to the visit.

We may like to think that what we do is *the* major factor influencing the health of a pregnancy. If so, we delude ourselves. What the mother does, or does not do, has a far greater effect on the outcome than any input by us. The very least we can do to acknowledge this is to provide a column in the notes where she can write things like 'Sickness better' or 'Feel awful' or 'Had scan today. What does excess liquor mean?' or 'Damian has chicken-pox I'm shattered' or 'Fags down to 3 per day' or 'Booked NCT classes'. And there is the great joy in recording 'Felt first movements today'.

THE 'MINOR' DISORDERS OF PREGNANCY

We are often consulted about the discomforts and disorders of pregnancy and here our knowledge of the woman's home circumstances can be of help.

Nausea and vomiting

There are many theories current about the causes of nausea in early pregnancy.

Masson, Anthony and Chau conclude from their study published in the *British Journal of Gynaecology and Obstetrics* (Vol. 92, no. 3, pp. 221–5) that serum chorionic gonadotrophin is the hormone mainly responsible for the condition, while reports from Sweden find links with gallstones (*Doctor Magazine*, 28 November, 1985). Lack of vitamin B6 has also been suggested as a cause. The successful treatment of a case of severe nausea of pregnancy by injection of vitamin B6, 100 mgm fortnightly, is described by a woman in the AIMS journal of winter 1986/87. The theory is postulated that in some women the condition is caused by a congenital inability to absorb B6 from the gastro-intestinal tract. Psychological reasons, such as fear of pregnancy, immaturity, attention-seeking have been advanced as reasons by some practitioners. (It is interesting to note that these misogynistic theories are usually expressed by male, or nulliparous female, persons.)

As the causes are legion so also have been the remedies. Simple alkalis seem to be as effective as Maxalon (metoclopramide). Other remedies include sipping aerated waters of various flavours, the carminative effect brings some temporary relief. Many women find ginger beneficial, either in the form of a little pellet of root ginger scraped off with a sharp knife and sucked or as ginger ale. Interestingly there is a reference in the *Lancet* (20 March, 1982) to the use of powdered ginger in the treatment of motion sickness, and there is a description of a successful treatment of a severe case of hyperemesis gravidarum with ginger capsules in the

California Association of Midwives' Newsletter (January 1985, p. 2).

Sometimes we can help the woman identify that changing her diet may be beneficial. 'Junk' food should be eliminated. An excellent leaflet *Nausea and Vomiting in Early Pregnancy* can be obtained from Dr B. M. Pickard, Lane End Farm, Dewton, Ilkley, Yorks, LFZ 90HP.

Backache

Backache is a common complaint during pregnancy. If the midwife has visited the home she will know what the kitchen is like: things such as the height of work surfaces make a difference. The height of the washing-up bowl can be raised by putting it on top of an upturned baking dish in the sink. If the worktop or sink is too high a duck board can be used to stand on. A mother with backache should be persuaded to give up standing at an ironing board. If her partner cannot take over this job, she should really cut down the family ironing or learn to do it sitting down.

What type of bed does she have? An interior sprung mattress bought at the time of marriage can have become a soft, sagging backache-producer, four babies and ten years later. Here a stiff board under the mattress can make an enormous difference. We can ask what is her favourite chair? If it is a low soft foam armchair it can be suggested that she change to a firmer more upright chair with a supportive cushion at the back.

If the woman's abdominal muscles are weak due to frequent pregnancies this can cause backache as she attempts to adjust to the changes in her centre of gravity. Many women with this problem benefit from wearing an abdominal support. Several types available from retailers of mother and baby requisites are both inexpensive and comfortable.

The woman may need help with her posture, a book balanced on her head may help her to stand tall, and a session with the physiotherapist in the local hospital can be really beneficial, especially if the physiotherapist is obstetrically trained.

If the mother is a very meticulous housewife it is unlikely that she will be happy to change her ways dramatically, despite her backache, but it is worth discussing with her ways of lessening her workload, and during the pregnancy sharing more of the household chores with her partner. It is useful to remind her that it will be difficult to try to be the district's best housewife as well as trying to be the world's best Mum. This is important because many first-time mothers set themselves quite unrealistic standards and can become very depressed when they cannot match the perfect mother image they have aimed for.

Varicose veins

The woman with varicose veins will almost certainly have been provided with support stockings by her GP or clinic, but is she wearing them? If not, why not? Maybe they do not fit properly. There is such a range of support tights and stockings available now, that she should not have to wear uncomfortable or unattractive ones. While support stockings are available on prescription by GPs, tights may only be obtained at present through the hospital antenatal clinics. Again we should ask about her favourite chair and recommend that she avoid sitting in a chair that has a hard ridge at the front just behind the knees, and we should be reminding her to get the family to help her to remember not to sit with her legs crossed. The woman with varicose veins is at greater risk of deep venous thrombosis and we should mention that the midwife or GP should be informed if there is any swelling or calf pain in the affected leg.

Cramp

Many women will complain of cramp during pregnancy. The favourite site for this seems to be the calf muscles, and it typically attacks in the very early morning. The woman turns over in her sleep and is suddenly woken by the severe pain of her calf muscles in spasm. Or it can occur when she first wakes and moves to get out of bed. This can almost always be alleviated, if not cured, by increasing the woman's calcium intake just before she retires to bed, e.g. with a milky drink with some added dried skimmed milk powder, or some cottage cheese, or yoghurt. If the woman cannot tolerate or dislikes dairy produce, her general practitioner can be asked to prescribe calcium tablets. The mechanism appears to be that the maternal blood calcium levels fall during the night, as the growing baby takes calcium from the mother, and this fall is enough to cause the cramp.

Thrush

Thrush can be a nuisance throughout life but pregnancy can exacerbate the condition. We can give general hygiene advice and stress the importance of avoiding the warm, moist, enclosed vulval environments (e.g. tight-fitting nylon pants under nylon tights under stretch jeans) that predispose to the condition. Cotton pants and either open-crutch tights or stockings help, and going around at home without under-wear can be suggested. Other remedies for this condition include live yoghurt as a topical application to the vulval area and the careful insertion into the vagina of a tampon or sponge soaked in natural yoghurt and left *in situ* overnight. Eating a carton of live yoghurt daily can also be recommended. In places like London where the water is very alkaline, the midwife can suggest bathing the vulval area with water made acid with the addition of vinegar to the bath or bowl. If the condition does not respond to these simple measures, treatment with an antimonilial agent is probably required and we should refer to the GP, because at the time of writing a midwife may not prescribe for this condition. Interestingly, the woman can buy an antimonilial agent such as Canestean ointment over the counter from a chemist, but it is cheaper to go to the GP and obtain a prescription for it.

Urinary tract infections

Some women experience frequent attacks of cystitis, and this condition is worsened by pregnancy. Many treat themselves by drinking large amounts of water, lemon barley or aerated water. Even if this treatment causes abatement of symptoms it is still very important for the future health of the woman's urinary system that bacteriological examination is made of a midstream specimen of urine, and an appropriate antibiotic advised if a significant bacteriuria is present. This will require referral to the general practitioner for prescription.

We should ensure that the woman understands how to produce a midstream specimen of urine and realises the importance of finishing any course of antibiotics that have been prescribed. We should tell her she should not hesitate to call if the condition does not respond to the treatment prescribed.

General advice shoud be given about the continued importance of a good fluid intake, and a short explanation about why urinary tract infections are common in pregnancy is often appreciated. Women who suffer from cystitis will find great help and comfort from reading Angela Kilmartin's book *Understanding Cystitis: A Complete Self-help Guide*.

Stress incontinence

This is one of the most miserable 'minor' disorders of pregnancy. The mother may have been told that it is not serious and that it will improve after the birth, but that does not help her *now*. Exercises are of limited value because so much of the condition is caused by the increased levels of progesterone and it is not going to get better as the pregnancy progresses. The last few weeks can be a real misery for many women – afraid to watch a comedy programme, afraid that a sneeze at an inopportune moment will result in an embarrassing spurt. The use of baby disposable nappies tucked into snugly-fitting pants can be a godsend. The waterproof backing prevents the awful threat of a wet skirt or chair. Even the very small size can cope with the amount of urine lost at a 'stress'.

Iron deficiency anaemia of pregnancy

There is a considerable difference of medical opinion and advice concerning the routine prophylactic prescription of iron supplements in pregnancy to healthy women eating a nutritionally adequate diet. There have been many studies reported in the medical journals both advocating and abnegating the practice. On the one hand there is the evidence that total body iron stores fall in pregnancy, and that the fall in haemoglobin levels cannot just be attributed to the hypervolaemia of pregnancy, and therefore routine administration of iron is beneficial. The contrary view is that in the presence of haemoglobin levels that are within the normal range, the oral administration of iron salts, e.g. ferrous fumarate, ferrous gluconate, or ferrous sulphate is ineffective, as very little of the amount swallowed will be absorbed through the digestive tract. There is also the view that the administration of iron interferes with the absorption of other equally valuable minerals, e.g. zinc. It is certainly the experience of many midwives that iron tablets do cause digestive disturbances, either constipation or colicky pain and loose stools, and aggravate nausea. Where a woman is routinely prescribed iron, the differences in medical opinion should be explained to her in language that she can understand and the decision of whether or not to take routine iron supplements should be hers.

Where iron deficiency anaemia exists the situation is different, and of course midwives will be aware that iron deficiency anaemia is not diagnosed on the haemoglobin levels alone but on a careful examination of the blood picture as a whole. Many midwives find it useful to keep a list of the normal haematological values of pregnant women in the antenatal bag. This condition does require treatment. The midwife should talk to the woman about diet, discussing with her the iron-rich foods that she finds acceptable, and can afford. The diet should also include adequate amounts of vitamin C and folic acid to assist absorption. The woman should be encouraged to take the iron prescribed, and if it causes digestive upset to tell the prescriber so that an alternative can be tried. Occasionally liquid iron preparations are better tolerated. There are several vegetable-based iron preparations available which may be more acceptable to some women.

THE 'MAJOR DISORDER' OF PREGNANCY:
PRE-ECLAMPSIA

Mild pre-eclampsia is a fairly common occurrence in our society. The community midwife will see many cases of pre-eclampsia of varying severity in her practice. As this is a deviation from normal the involvement of a medical practitioner is mandatory, but the midwife will be asked to visit and monitor the milder cases at home. Important factors to bear in mind are the age, gestation, history, and parity of the woman, and her social and domestic circumstances.

The following is a useful method of scoring risk factors in pre-eclampsia. A score of 3 or more should be recorded as significant.

- AGE   Pregnant women under 18 and the over 40. Score 1 if either factor present.
- GESTATION   The under-32 weeks and the post-term pregnancy. Score 1 if either factor present.
- HISTORY   A history of the condition in previous pregnancies. Score 1.
- PARITY   Primigravidae. Score 2.
- SOCIAL CIRCUMSTANCES   A mother unsupported by husband, partner, family or friends. Score 1.

In the latter weeks of pregnancy the midwife will be seeing the woman at frequent intervals and may be caring for and checking on the cases of mild pre-eclampsia. These cases will either have been diagnosed by the midwife herself during her care or referred to her by the general practitioner or hospital clinic. It is wise to discuss all cases of pre-eclampsia with either the general practitioner obstetrician or the hospital obstetrician. Usually the treatment of a mild case is rest at home for the mother, and vigilant inactivity on the part of the midwife, but mild pre-eclampsia with a score of 6 risk factors obviously requires further thought about the need for hospital care. And of course any mild pre-eclampsia can become severe pre-eclampsia and require medical intervention. A useful guide path can be:

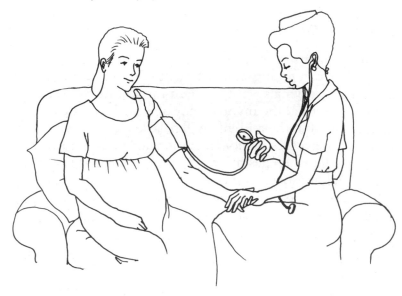

Mild pre-eclampsia

Slight rise in blood pressure from previous levels with some oedema, weight gain greater than usual, no albuminuria, risk factors less than 3. Treatment: rest. Check every other day by midwife. Woman instructed to call if any headache, visual disturbances, abdominal pain, sickness.

Outcomes

1 *Blood pressure returns to former levels, oedema less.* Report to GP or obstetrician, reduce frequency of visits.
2 *No change.* Continue regime, but check family support. Is she in fact resting? Can she rest? Check diet. Is she receiving enough protein in her diet? Brewer states that increasing the protein intake controls pre-eclampsia. Continue to visit every other day. Liaise with appropriate medical colleagues.
3 *The condition worsens.* BP continues to rise but the distolic is less than 100. The oedema increases slightly but the urine remains clear. This is the difficult one. To admit or not to admit? The risk factor score can be helpful. The

case should be discussed with either the GP or the medical staff of the hospital if the woman is planning a hospital birth. If a home birth has been planned the possibility of changing to a hospital birth should be discussed with the woman at this stage. If this has been a midwife's case with no medical involvement, now is the time to seek medical aid. Should there not be a general practitioner obstetrician in the area who is willing to attend, the midwife should seek the medical aid of the hospital staff. Should the decision be made to continue with domiciliary care, the midwife should visit daily or twice daily as she sees fit. The advice to the woman to call if she has any of the symptoms previously described should be reinforced. Some midwives give the woman or her partner reagent sticks to test for protein every time urine is passed and advise them to call if it becomes present.

4 *The blood pressure continues to rise, the diastolic is above 100, the oedema increases and there is protein present in a clean specimen of urine.* Urgent admission to a consultant maternity unit should be advised. Should the midwife think that there is a fulminating pre-eclampsia present she should consider whether the admission should be by ambulance following sedation. The GP could be called to prescribe this. Whenever possible this should be discussed with the admitting hospital medical staff. Factors to take into consideration would be the distance to be travelled, and the likelihood of traffic hold-ups. Inner-city rush hour, or tourist coaches in rural lanes at peak holiday times, can both cause delays.

Should severe frontal headache, epigastric pain and/or visual disturbances be present the possibility of admission via the obstetric emergency service (The Flying Squad) should be considered. Community midwives will get to know their local facilities and the views on this subject held by the consultant obstetrician to whom she and/or the general practitioner is referring the case.

If we have to admit a pregnant woman as an emergency we

should consider that there may be children expected home from school, or little children to be met from school. There could also be dependant relatives or the welfare of pets to be considered. The midwife may be able to assist in contacting friends or relatives to help, or she may need to enlist the help of the health visitor, or the local Social Services Department.

Whether it be giving advice about deworming the dog, or helping to arrange the transfer of a fulminating pre-eclampsia, it is the duty and role of the community midwife to combine her theoretical and practical midwifery skills with a knowledge of the domestic, social and environmental circumstances of the women to whom she is offering care in pregnancy.

References

AIMS Journal. Winter 1986/7.

Ball, Jean A. (1987). *Reactions to Motherhood: The Role of Post-natal Care*. Cambridge: Cambridge University Press.

Brewer, Thomas H. (1982). *Metabolic Toxaemia of Late Pregnancy*. New Canaan, Connecticut: Keats Publishing Inc.

California Association of Midwives Newsletter, January 1985, p. 2.

Doctor Magazine. 28 November, 1985.

Elliot, Rose (1984, new ed. 1988). *Vegetarian Mother and Baby Book*, London: Fontana.

Kilmartin, Angela (1980). *Understanding Cystitis. A Complete Self-help Guide*. London: Arrow Books.

Kilmartin, Angela (1986). *Victims of Thrush and Cystitis*. London: Arrow Books.

Lancet. March 20 1982.

Masson, Anthony and Chau. British Journal of Gynaecology and Obstetrics **92**, 3, pp. 221–5.

Royal College of Obstetricians and Gynaecologists. Report of the R.C.O.G. working party on antenatal and intrapartum care. (1982). Royal College of Obstetrics and Gynaecology, 27 Sussex Place, Regent's Park, London NW1 4RG.

Chapter Three

The Community Midwife Working in Hospital

The 'domiciliary in and out' scheme (domino delivery) has been hailed for years as the answer to many of the ills in the maternity services. Despite this, the scheme has never really taken off and in 1981 only 3.6% of women actually had a domino delivery (DHSS, 1987). It is likely that only a tiny proportion of those women will actually have met their midwife before labour, much less have been able to form a relationship with her. This is a pity for a properly organised domino delivery can be very satisfying for women, and for midwives it can be a way of utilising all our skills and providing appropriate care for individual women, as the concept is based on the woman knowing her midwives and having much of her labour care in her own home. The relationship between the woman and the midwife is built up during pregnancy when the midwife does much of the woman's antenatal care, usually in partnership with the woman's GP.

When she goes into labour the woman contacts her midwife, who comes to her home, decides whether she is in established labour, assesses how she is progressing and advises her accordingly. When the time is right the woman (and her partner/other children/friend) and the midwife go to the hospital, where the midwife looks after her in labour and delivers her baby. About six hours later they all 'transfer back' to the woman's home (either by car or by ambulance) where the woman's care is continued by her midwife or midwives twice daily for the first three days and then once a day until the tenth day, and then as necessary until the baby is four weeks old.

Domino deliveries can be flexible enough to cater for individual women's needs, as is shown in the following case histories.

ANNA

Anna, a primigravida of 37, who lived 14 miles from the hospital, booked for a domino delivery. During Anna's pregnancy she had seven of her antenatal checks by her local midwives – Ruth, Chandra and Clarice. She had met all three midwives at least twice each and she felt she knew Clarice especially well because she had been to the classes which were Clarice's particular interest and responsibility. Anna's pregnancy had been uneventful, except that at 37 weeks her blood pressure had risen from its usual 110/60 to 120/80. Ruth, who was seeing her that day, checked on Anna's diet and encouraged Anna to eat more protein. She discovered that Anna had been busy for the preceding two weeks and hadn't eaten properly, so encouraged her to have two pints of milk, two eggs and two servings of meat or fish each day with fresh fruit and vegetables (Brewer, 1982) and to rest for a couple of hours during the day. When Chandra visited Anna to check her blood pressure three days later it was back to normal.

At 39 weeks and two days Anna began having contractions every 10 minutes, and she telephoned the on-call midwife who was Clarice. Clarice ascertained whether Anna had had a 'show' (No), whether her membranes had ruptured (No), whether the baby had been active recently (Yes) and how often the contractions were coming (every 10 minutes). Clarice talked with Anna on the phone for several minutes to ascertain how she sounded while she was having a contraction and Clarice came to the conclusion that Anna was not in strong or established labour as she was able to talk to Clarice throughout her contractions. It was 6 a.m. so Clarice ascertained that she had time to have a shower and to fix her children's packed lunches before she left. When she arrived at Anna's flat at 9 a.m. Anna's contractions had reduced to every 20 minutes and were fading away. Clarice decided that this episode of contractions was due to the baby's head going down, wasn't true labour and would eventually subside. Anna's blood pressure was normal, the baby's heart was regular (128 beats per minute), so Clarice left Anna her bleep number so that Anna could contact her and rang Anna every few hours to see what was happening. Within four hours the contractions had completely died away and Anna resumed her normal life.

Anna was terribly apologetic for having called Clarice unnecessarily, but Clarice reassured her that most women seem to call their midwives out on a false alarm at least once before true labour starts – almost as if they are testing the system to make sure it works. Many women go into hospital at least once prior to proper labour being established and many women call their midwife at least once before they go into established labour at a home delivery.

Anna carried on seeing her three midwives at her antenatal visits. At 41 weeks plus four days Anna bleeped the midwife on call that day, who was Ruth. Anna had had a show, it was 4 a.m. and she had been contracting since midnight. Ruth asked her the usual questions about whether her waters had gone, whether the baby had been moving recently. It became obvious as they talked that when Anna had a contraction it was strong enough to cause her to stop talking and breathe in panting breaths.

Ruth said that she would be at Anna's flat as quickly as she could. She asked Anna to put on all the lights in the front of the flat so that she could identify it easily. Ruth arrived at Anna's flat at 4.55 a.m. and greeted Phil and Anna. Phil offered to make a cup of tea and Ruth watched Anna while she sipped her tea, noticing how she was coping with contractions. This enabled her to build up an idea of how strong the contractions were. She also felt Anna's abdomen during a couple of contractions. Then she palpated Anna's abdomen and listened to the baby's heart, took Anna's temperature, pulse and blood pressure and asked her to pass urine, which Ruth then checked. She asked Anna to wash herself in her vulval area, donned sterile gloves and examined Anna vaginally.

Findings on vaginal examination were: vulva and vagina warm and moist; cervix 50% effaced, 4 cm dilated, central, soft but well applied to presenting part; presenting part cephalic, head 1 cm above ischial spines.

The labour was progressing well, Anna was well relaxed and coping well with contractions, she leaned forward against the kitchen work surface or against the kitchen table during each contraction for a couple of hours, then she spent about an hour and a half in the bath. When Ruth did the next vaginal examination Anna was 7 cm dilated, so she rang the hospital and told them that she was bringing Anna in for a domino delivery. She made sure that there was some heating on in the bedroom ready for their return. They packed some sandwiches and Phil drove to the hospital with Anna sitting in the back of the car, and Ruth following in her own car. When they arrived at the hospital, Ruth took Anna and Phil up to the labour ward and they settled down in the room which had been allocated to them.

Ruth carried on her documentation in the notes which Anna had carried ever since booking for a domino delivery. Anna progressed well in labour, using Entonox for the relief of her pain towards the end of her first stage, and at 2 p.m. she was finally overwhelmed with an urge to push. Baby Derek emerged at 2.30 p.m. He had an Apgar score of 9:10:10 and was a lusty little boy of 7 lb 6 oz (3.3 kg). Anna had a graze on her perineum but she didn't require any suturing.

After Derek had suckled and all three adults had had a cup of tea and a sandwich and Clarice (who was in the hospital) had been in to see how Ruth was feeling and whether she wanted some help or a meal break, Ruth washed and dressed Derek, then took Anna to the bath and by 6.30 p.m. they were all ready to go home, four hours after the birth. Anna and Derek went down to the car in a wheelchair and sat in the back. Having helped Anna into the flat and into bed, Ruth snuggled Derek down by his mother, told them that

Chandra would visit them first thing in the morning, and in the meantime made sure that they had the midwives' phone number handy.

In the morning Chandra informed Anna's GP of Derek's birth and he came to examine the baby. Anna had enjoyed the birth, she enjoyed having someone with her who she knew, and she had plenty of rest afterwards, sleeping in her own bed in her own bedroom. Phil was able to be involved in the care of his baby from the very start of the baby's life and the couple treasured this very much.

ESTELLE

Estelle was expecting her third baby, she had had three 'false alarms' and was beginning to be very embarrassed every time she rang the midwives. She finally called Chandra at 11 p.m. on a Sunday evening. When Chandra spoke to Estelle on the phone it was obvious that she was in strong, established labour. Chandra said that Estelle should come immediately to the hospital and that Chandra would meet her in the delivery room.

Estelle and Chandra met up at 11.45 p.m. and baby Kirsty was born 30 minutes later. By the time Chandra had washed the baby and taken Estelle to have a bath and finished her notes it was 3.15 a.m. They decided that it was silly to go home at that time and Estelle stayed in the postnatal ward overnight and went home in her husband's car at 11.30 the following morning. Clarice visited her an hour later.

GLORIA

Gloria's labour was slightly more complicated. She was a primigravida whose membranes ruptured spontaneously at 40 weeks at 2 a.m. She bleeped the on-call midwife, who was Clarice. Clarice came round to find that Gloria was having no contractions. When Clarice had ascertained that Gloria was not having contractions, that the fetal heart was good, that Gloria's condition was healthy, that the baby's head was engaged and there had been no cord prolapse, she suggested that Gloria should go to bed and try to sleep.

Gloria woke at 8.30 a.m., still with no contractions. Ruth was on call the following day so she visited Gloria to check the fetal heart at 9 a.m., 1.30 p.m., 5 p.m. and again at 9 p.m. She was woken at midnight by Gloria bleeping her, she was having contractions every five minutes.

Ruth went to Gloria's house and looked after her at home until 4 cm dilatation, when Gloria decided that she wanted to go into hospital and have an epidural. They went to the hospital and Gloria had an epidural which seemed to slow down her labour. After consultation with the hospital registrar, Syntocinon was put up and Gloria became fully dilated at 12 midday. Clarice had taken over in the morning when her on-call duty began and stayed with Gloria for her normal delivery of a little girl, Rosene. Five hours after Rosene's birth, Gloria felt active and ready to go home. She was checked to make sure that the effects of her epidural had fully worn off and she went home by car with her boyfriend and the midwife following.

Once home Gloria and Rosene were put into bed together and they started life together in their own home. Ralph, Gloria's boyfriend, was truly involved from the start, needing to provide all the food for the next few days and enabled to feel really useful.

JOAN

Joan needed a caesarean section. She went into hospital at 5 cm dilatation after an extremely long labour with a posterior-positioned baby. The baby showed signs of fetal distress and Clarice, who was with her, consulted the obstetric registrar, who on the results of fetal blood sampling advised that a caesarean section was the delivery of choice for this baby. Joan and Gareth, her husband, agreed and Joan had a caesarean section. Clarice was with Joan and she 'took' the baby at the caesarean section, and carried her out very quickly to meet her father. After the operation Clarice took some photographs of baby Holly as she met her sleepy mother for the first time. Joan felt exhausted for several days after the 'section', and she was also in considerable pain. She stayed in hospital for five days with her midwives coming in each day to help with her postnatal care. When she went home on Day 5 Chandra arranged to be at her home half an hour after she arrived, and made sure that Joan went to bed. Chandra arranged a nappy-changing place for Holly, made sure Gareth was able to cope with all that he had to do, and suggested that when Gareth went back to work Joan's twin sister might be asked to come over each day and help Joan.

All these domino deliveries were adapted to meet each woman's particular needs. Each woman had a midwife she knew antenatally with her during early labour at home, later in labour in hospital, then caring for her and her baby post-natally in hospital in conjunction with hospital staff and/or at home.

HOME ASSESSMENT OF LABOUR

The value for women and their babies of being visited at home and assessed there by community midwives was underlined by Klein and colleagues (1983) in a paper printed in the *British Journal of Obstetrics and Gynaecology*. This describes a study of 252 women in a randomised trial. Sixty-three primigravid and 63 multigravid women were booked for shared care with their GPs but for delivery in the consultant unit; 63 primigravid women and 63 multigravid were booked for GP unit care. (By GP unit was actually meant whichever of the labour wards in the consultant unit the community midwife was using in conjunction with the GP, thus today it could be room 9 and tomorrow it could be rooms 3 and 8.) The basic difference between the two groups was in their treatment in early labour. Women having shared care telephoned the labour ward when they started labour and were advised from there. Women having GP deliveries telephoned the community midwife or the GP when they started labour. Sixty-two per cent of the primigravid women and 33% of the multigravid women were assessed in early labour at home by the community midwife, and 22% of the multigravid women were assessed in early labour at their GP's surgery.

The differences for the women and their babies was highly significant. Despite the fact that women booked for GP unit deliveries had longer labours, they spent much less time in the hospital before delivery than did the women having shared care. They needed less pain relief during labour, had less intervention, less fetal monitoring, less augmentation with Syntocinon, fewer instrumental deliveries, and their babies needed less resuscitation. All these favourable outcomes presumably derived from the fact that these women were assessed in labour at home by a midwife, and the fact that more women having shared care were admitted to the labour ward in false labour (22% of the primigravid women and 12% of the multigravid women).

Klein *et al.* comment, 'the difficulty of the shared care system for those women at low risk may be that they are grouped with high-risk women, and there is the natural tendency for high-risk care to spill over into their management'.

There are other studies which show the value of community care by midwives which are enumerated in this book.

Women who are not booked for domino delivery but who are intending to stay in hospital could also have labour care at home in early labour provided by the community midwife. For example, take the woman who telephones to say that her membranes have ruptured but who has no contractions. How much more pleasant it is (and how much less risk of infection there is) if the midwife goes round to her home, checks on the liquor to make sure that it does not contain meconium, palpates the abdomen to ensure that the fetal head is engaged and listens to the fetal heart for a couple of minutes to preclude cord prolapse, and suggests that the woman can continue as usual until she goes into labour. This she is likely to do within 24 hours, according to the trial carried out in Bristol and reported by Conway *et al.* in the *American Journal of Obstetrics and Gynecology* in 1984, and according to Varner and Galask in the *American Journal of Obstetrics and Gynecology* in 1981.

The midwife can keep an eye on the woman by popping in from time to time through the day whilst the woman in her own home is at less risk of infection, is under less stress, can keep herself well nourished, and is more likely to go into normal physiological labour than if she is under stress in the hospital 'waiting' for something to happen. At home she can be catching up with the ironing, finishing painting the nursery, reading a good book, watching the television, having a leisurely bath, walking in the nearby park, writing letters, ringing her Mum, having coffee with friends – all with a delicious anticipation of excitements to come.

CLEMENTINE

Consider the following hypothetical situation. Clementine is booked for a hospital delivery and is having contractions. She just wants to know whether it is time for her to go in yet. Usually if a woman needs to ask it is too early, but how much more reassuring (and how much safer) for midwife Oona to visit her at home, watch Clementine while they sip a cup of tea, take Clementine's temperature, pulse and blood pressure, test her urine, palpate her abdomen, listen to the baby's heart, do or not do a vaginal examination and pronounce whether she thinks Clementine is in established labour yet. We have seen from the work of Klein and his colleagues, that women appear to fare better if they are kept out of hospital until they are in truly established labour, and one of the basic tenets of O'Driscoll is that no woman should be in the labour ward unless she is in established labour (O'Driscoll and Meagher, 1980).

Clementine can stay at home for longer than she would have done had she had no one to consult at home, she can go into hospital when she is in established labour, she can be delivered on the labour ward, Oona can pop in and see her if that is convenient. When she goes to the postnatal ward Oona can either pop in and see her, or wait until she comes home, when, as the local midwife she will be doing Clementine's postnatal care.

WORKING WITH HOSPITAL STAFF

In general

Community midwives spend most of their time in the community, either giving antenatal, delivery or postnatal care – but, as we have seen from the description of domino deliveries, they can do quite a significant amount of their care within the hospital, for which they will need to liaise with and rely upon the midwives and doctors who work there.

The community midwife can become a resource person for the hospital staff – with articles of interest, with local knowledge of breastfeeding counsellors, postnatal support groups, facilities in local shops. The community midwife can make sure that she takes part in hospital life with her colleagues – she can go to journal clubs, ethics groups, perinatal mortality meetings. Indeed, she can set up midwife support groups or journal clubs herself.

Working in a team

When midwives are working in a team (more about this in Chapter 13) and providing nearly all antenatal, delivery and postnatal care, they may be working inside the hospital because their 'patch' is around the hospital or they may be based inside a health or community centre. For antenatal consultations they will need one room which contains a sink, a couch and three chairs. A desk or table is also handy, and scales make the whole venue perfect.

The midwives working in such a team either visit women at home antenatally, and/or assess the woman at home in early labour, and then stay with her or pop in from time to time, as the situation warrants. A midwife can accompany the woman to hospital for delivery and then transfer her to

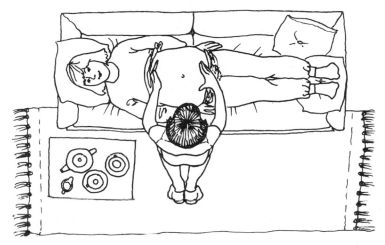

the postnatal ward or straight home. Any of the team can visit her while she is in the postnatal ward, to do her post-natal checks, show her how to bath her baby and change its nappy, take out her sutures if necessary, encourage her post-natal exercises and oversee her feeding of her baby. The same midwives can then offer care to the woman when she arrives home.

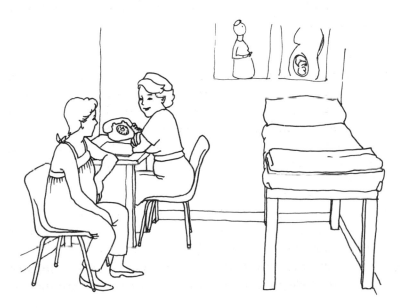

Forming a productive relationship with hospital staff

What does the community midwife need to do in order to
have the best and most productive relationship possible with
the staff in hospital? She needs to know them, and they need
to know her, by sight. She needs to talk with them frequently
and to be open and to invite them to come and see her world.
It can make a huge difference to a hospital midwife's attitude
to community midwives if she has spent a morning with them
and has been able to get to know them and how they work. As
mentioned on p. 44, the community midwife can act as a resource about what is going on in the local community – bringing press cuttings of interest from local papers for the staff to
see, or articles of general midwifery interest that she has
culled from the magazines she persuades the GPs to give her.

If the community midwives hold their own antenatal clinic
within the hospital antenatal clinic they need to discuss with
the antenatal clinic sister what level of facilities they will be
able to have. They need to ascertain how they will get hold of
blood results and where results are stored. Presumably all
women will be carrying their own notes, but a tiny minority
may want theirs kept within the hospital. The community
midwives need to discuss this with the antenatal clinic sister
and the records clerks for the maternity department. It is important for the community midwives to be as friendly and
loyal to the hospital midwives as possible: the smoother the
working relationship, the more satisfying it is for both
groups and the more pleasant it is for the women.

Working alongside hospital staff in the delivery ward

When the community midwife is working within the delivery
ward in the hospital there are certain golden rules to follow:

- Telephone the labour ward before you bring in a woman
  who is in labour. Let whoever you speak to, know that you
  will be accompanying her. If the couple are in agreement,
  offer to have a student with you.
- Greet everyone and introduce yourself when you go into
  the delivery ward, also introduce the labouring couple.

- Greet the registrar on duty, tell him (*sic*) what has happened so far. Assure him that you will let him know in good time if there is anything that you need him for, but at the moment everything is progressing normally.

- If you need to give any drugs use the hospital drugs and drug book and abide by the drug policy, remembering that you can always give *less* than is suggested as long as you write it in the notes, the drug book and the register.

- Put the birth in the hospital birth register even if you put it into your own register too. Remember to send in the birth notification.

- Come to an agreement with the sister-in-charge about clearing up after the delivery. She may be content if you clear away the trollies and soiled linen and wash down the delivery bed, but on the other hand she may expect you to restock the cupboards and make up the bed. Tell her what else you have to do and be grateful for her help.

- Liaise with the obstetric registrar but always be pleasant to the SHO and offer to show him things that may be useful to him – such as suturing, delivery in an alternative position, or setting up the room to allow greater freedom of movement for the woman.

- If highly technical equipment is needed that you don't know how to operate, such as fetal blood sampling or the setting up of an epidural, ask another midwife for help or tell the doctor you are working with that you are unfamiliar with this procedure, so would he help you? He would feel just as frightened if he were thrust into a home delivery or if he suddenly had to do open heart surgery or stripping of varicose veins.

- You cannot know where everything is kept in the labour ward, don't be embarrassed to ask and don't be hard on yourself if you then can't remember another time. Remember that your confusion is very good for the labour ward staff, who tend to look upon the labour ward as 'home' and forget how intimidating it is for new staff – much less for mothers and fathers!

- Depending on your 'patch', you may always liaise with the

obstetric registrar or in some areas you may be expected to liaise with the GP. In hospital, insist that you liaise with the registrar. The houseman is there as a learner and you should be teaching him as much as you can. He is not there for you to consult, his knowledge level is just not adequate, but if you go out of your way to help him to learn you will be able to influence his practice for ever.

In the postnatal ward

In the postnatal ward it is important that the community midwife learns about the specific forms that have to be filled in when performing Guthrie tests on a baby in hospital, or when transferring a woman from hospital to home. She often sees the paperwork with new eyes, and can thus sometimes be a source of change in that she can suggest simpler systems (paperwork tends to be more streamlined in the community). She needs to let the postnatal ward staff know whether she has just popped in for a 'social' call on the woman or whether she is here to help them and will carry out a post-natal check – or baby bath, or top and tail demonstration.

The other role that midwives tend to be too timid to take on is that of giving guidance to the doctors. If you are unhappy with anything a doctor does or the way he addresses a woman it is essential that you should speak to him about it – otherwise he cannot learn, He needs to de-velop an awareness that what he does *matters* – especially to this woman, whose only mouthpiece may be her midwife.

A PLEA FOR CONTINUITY OF CARE

How babies are born and how women give birth are the very pivot of our culture. Women have been asking for the same people to be involved in their care all through pregnancy, labour and the postnatal period for years (see page 6). Women want and need us to provide continuity of care – when we make no effort to provide this it signifies that we are not listening to our clients and we are not providing the ser-vice they are asking for. We all work hard enough; it is pointless to work so hard and yet provide a service which is not the service women need from us. By making organisational changes we can provide continuity of care by a small group of midwives (the ideal of one or two midwives is not attainable yet), and the most rational place for this type of care to start is near to home – in the community.

References

Brewer, Thomas H. (1982). *Metabolic Toxaemia of Late Pregnancy*. New Canaan, Connecticut: Keats Publishing Inc.

Conway, D., Prendeville, W., Morris, A., Speller, D., Stirrat, G. (1984). Management of spontaneous rupture of the membranes in the absence of labour in primigravid women at term. *American Journal of Obstetrics and Gynecology*; 150: 947–51.

DHSS. (1987). Health and Personal Social Services Statistics for England 1987. Table VIII, Maternity and Child Health and Social Services, HMSO.

Durward, Lyn. (1983). Birth in Britain. *Parents*; 92 (November).

Flint, Caroline and Poulengeris, Polly. (1987). *The Know Your Midwife Report*. London. Heinemann.

Klein, M., Lloyd, I., Redman, C., Bull, M., Turnbull, A. C. (1983). A comparison of low-risk pregnant women booked for delivery in two systems of care: shared care (consultant) and integrated general practice unit. *British Journal of Obstetrics and Gynaecology*; 90: 118–28 (February).

Micklethwait, L., Beard, R., Shaw, K. (1978). Expectations of a pregnant woman in relation to her treatment. *British Medical Journal*; 2: 188–91.

O'Driscoll, Kieran, Meagher, Declan. (1980). *Active Management of Labour*. London, Philadelphia and Toronto: W. B. Saunders.

Royal College of Obstetricians and Gynaecologists. (1982). *Report of the RCOG working party on antenatal and intrapartum care*. Royal College of Obstetrics and Gynaecology, 27 Sussex Place, Regent's Park, London NW1 4RG.

Varner, M. W. and Galask, R. P. (1981). Conservative management of premature rupture of the membranes. *American Journal of Obstetrics and Gynecology*; 140: 39–45.

Chapter Four

Births at Home

Babies have always been born at home. This seems such an obvious statement to make. Every midwife knows in her head that it is only in the last thirty years or so that most babies have been born away from their homes, and, as has been said in our first chapter, we now have research evidence that points to the restoration of birth at home as a safe option for many women, who have homes, and who wish to give birth there.

Home births can safely take place in inner city 'squats' and in stately country homes and in every sort of habitation in between. So what do we need? What do the parents need to get ready? How do we organise it all?

We need:
- A reasonably clean room.
- A source of clean hot and cold water.
- Availability of good light, remembering that we may need to suture the perineum (an anglepoise lamp is excellent, but a bedside lamp with the shade removed can be held by an assistant). A good big torch is also quite adequate. Years ago suturings in the district were done with the front light from the midwife's bike, but that option isn't available now that we all have cars!
- A reliable method of heating the room we plan to use. If the only method of heating is electricity in an area prone to power cuts it is useful to have a second source of heat available. Portable Calor gas heaters can be borrowed from Social Services Departments in some areas. If the heating (and light) is dependent on an electric slot meter, we must really stress to the parents the importance of having a large supply of the correct coins available.
- Attendants willing and able to provide support during labour and to undertake responsibility for the domestic

duties for at least one, ideally two weeks, following the birth. The local authority may be able to provide home help either at a nominal charge, if the family income is low, or at cost price.

- Adequate toilet facilities. What one person considers 'adequate' may be described as primitive by another. The midwife needs to ensure that the woman can wash her vulva and perineal area in a comfortable and hygienic manner postnatally, following micturition and defecation. This can be done in the bidet in an en suite luxury bathroom, or can be done over a commode, bedpan, or bucket with two jugs, one of clean soapy water and one of clean rinsing water. If a woman lives in a home without a bathroom and normally keeps herself clean she will continue to do so using the facilities she has. The midwife may think that the woman would be more comfortable in hospital, and may indeed advise this, but it is perfectly possible to maintain good hygiene without a bathroom, although it requires ingenuity, flexibility, and an understanding of the basic principles involved.
- A telephone in the house, or 24-hour access to one in a neighbouring house. It is not advisable to rely on public telephones being in working order. Fortunate midwives will have radio telephones.
- Ready access for an ambulance should it be necessary to transfer the woman to hospital in labour.

The home should not be more than half an hour away from a consultant maternity unit. Having said this, there may be occasions when a woman will elect to have a home birth despite living a distance from obstetric help. This of course will be her decision and the midwife's duty will be to ensure that it has been an accurately informed decision, and that she continues to give the woman her care and support.

Pregnant women approaching term often instinctively start 'nesting', preparing the house and getting things ready. Many midwives will arrange to make an extended evening visit to the home about the 37th/38th week of pregnancy so

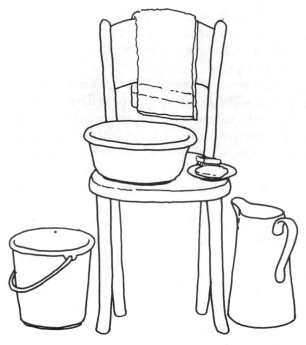

they can discuss with the parents the final preparations and make sure that all is ready.

The list of things that the woman should be asked to provide will vary according to individual needs and preferences but a possible check list could include the following:

- Soap, towel, and a new cheap nailbrush for the midwife's use.
- If the bathroom is some way from the planned birth room or if there isn't a bathroom, a plastic washing up bowl, a saucer for the soap and nailbrush, a jug to carry water and a slop bucket should be requested. This can all be arranged on a chair. The family heirloom of great grannie's beautiful old ewer and basin, however aesthetically pleasing, is to be avoided for the sake of the midwife's nerves!
- Two surfaces, e.g. small table, top of a chest-of-drawers, bedside cabinet, dressing table. One is to set out the equipment for the birth, the other is to set out the things that

might be needed for the baby. Check the surfaces offered and if there is any danger of damage ask that they be covered with something waterproof. Not all parents want a permanent reminder of the birth in the form of water ringmarks on the Chippendale! Some midwives ask for two trays for the same purpose. This is particularly useful if the woman is unsure where she wants to give birth as the trays can easily be carried to beside the sofa, before the sitting-room fire, or back to her bedroom, or wherever she ends up.

- A waterproof covering for her bed, sofa, or carpet. Avoid thin plastic – it only gets crumpled up. A shower curtain, a plastic table cover, or a length of thick polythene are all suitable. A babies changing mat with an inco pad or towel on it is an ideal thing to put under the mother for the actual delivery; the trough shape of the mat contains the liquor, blood, and any other body fluids nicely. Our aim should be that the room should hold no permanent evidence that a birth has taken place there. The bed and floor should not be stained in any way if careful use has been made of inco pads.
- A roll of cotton wool. This can be rolled up into small balls and kept in a clean pillowslip or polythene bags.
- A box of tissues or a kitchen roll.
- A small bottle of whatever antiseptic the midwife prefers for vulval swabbing – or whatever the woman prefers. Some women will produce their own homeopathic lotions.
- A small bottle of almond or other nice-smelling light vegetable oil for backrubbing, baby massage, etc.
- A hot water bottle for warming the receiving blanket, and baby clothes, also for the woman to have for her back in labour and to be available afterwards, if as many women do, she gets the shivers just after the third stage is complete.
- Two nice soft receiving blankets for the baby. If the mother takes her baby into her arms immediately, it is nice to have something special to cover baby and mother warmly with. Occasionally baby will need some help to establish regular respirations and a warm soft cover to

conserve heat is essential if one has to take the baby away from the heat of the mother's body. Pieces of soft towelling or flannelette are ideal.

- Something loose and comfortable for the mother to wear in labour, preferably big loose cotton T shirts, or short cotton nighties. Suggest she puts aside a couple of suitable garments in which she will feel comfortable.

- A cardboard box and a couple of dustbin liners to line the box with. This is for the rubbish. Plan how it will be disposed of. In the country it is easy, most gardens have incinerators, but the community midwife in an urban area will have to make arrangements with her local hospital for the disposal of waste. Many older midwives will remember when almost all homes had lovely big coal fires and the placenta was ceremoniously wrapped in the pieces of tarred paper supplied in the delivery pack, and burned on the fire. Superstition said that if the placenta 'popped' while being burned a person in the room would be pregnant within the year. As birth was a neighbourhood event many a young woman has sidled into the room, ostensibly to see the baby, but whispered, 'Has the afterbirth gone yet? My Mammy told me to come . . . .'

- If one is working without supplied sterile packs ask for a saucepan with a lid, a pudding basin, and an old but uncracked cup which will fit inside the saucepan. In early labour boil the lot for twenty minutes with a quantity of cotton wool swabs. When cool this will give a sterilised bowl, sterilised galleypot, sterilised water, and sterile swabs.

- Two packets of large sanitary pads and a small packet of disposable napkins. Even if the woman plans to use towelling napkins for baby, they are extremely useful for the woman to use if the membranes rupture, and she wants to walk around.

- A spare 100-watt electric light bulb – because many years ago at a birth, second stage, head advancing nicely – the bulb went . . . Husband in a panic. Midwife said, 'Just put the landing light on.' He went out to the landing, got a chair, got up to the landing light to take the bulb out, over-

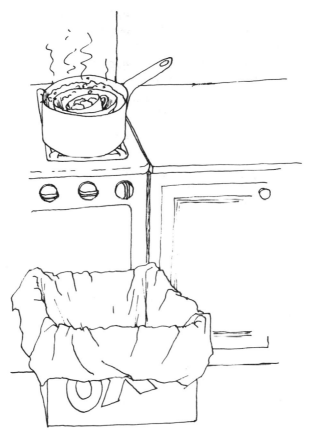

balanced, fell and broke his ankle. Midwife delivered the
baby by the light of a street lamp which was just outside
the window, then strapped up his ankle and sent for medical aid ... for him!

- A small jar of honey and a bottle of proprietary glucose
  drink, for the prevention and treatment of ketosis in a long
  labour or where the mother vomits in labour.
- Supply of baby clothes and baby toilet articles. Discussing
  and getting these ready with the mother can be the opportunity for parentcraft teaching about all sorts of things,
  concerning how babies should be dressed and cared for,
  and about the essentials and the luxury non-essentials.

Many women are happy to get together a layette of used

clothes and equipment from friends, relatives, and local jumble sales. The amount parents spend on their baby varies enormously and in some cases bears little relationship to what the midwife thinks the parents can afford. We must remember that for many parents in our society conspicuous expenditure on the expected baby is very important to them, and indicates their commitment. Nevertheless the midwife should give advice on wise spending if money is short.

It is important that we have prepared together for the labour and have discussed together the various positions that can be adopted for the actual birth. We should explain that the best-laid plans of women and midwives sometimes do not live up to expectations and that the position for birth in bed that felt good during our practice is awful at the actual event. Likewise the position in an Active Birth book that was fine when we practised it, turns out to be uncomfortable and lying on her back in bed is what feels best.

As we encourage the women to discuss with us what they think will be best for them, we should be honest and tell them of our weaknesses and strengths. If we prefer not to be behind a woman delivering on all fours and unable to see her face we should say so. She may still choose to deliver on all fours but we have been honest to each other about it. If we have arthritic knees and have difficulty on the floor we should say so too, and discuss how we can work together.

OUR EQUIPMENT

What do we carry with us in our little black bags or equivalent? Again there will be individual needs and variations, but the midwife setting out to attend home births should have:

Pinard's stethoscope
Portable fetal heart monitor
Sphygmomanometer
Urine-testing equipment

She will probably have these items together in an antenatal

bag as is described in Chapter 8. It is a good idea always to pack one's delivery bag in exactly the same way so that one can very quickly put one's hand on any item.

We will all pack our bags slightly differently but this is how a bag could be packed.

Right on top is a **small sterile paper sheet pack** and a **pair of gloves.**

Then a sealed, **sterile covered kidney dish** containing the instruments. They are sterilised by the hospital's Central Sterile Supply Department (CSSD).

The instruments are:

2 artery forceps. Kochers may be preferred to Spencer Wells by some midwives, because if the cord is clamped the toothed ends avoid the danger of the clamp slipping.

1 cord scissors
1 episiotomy scissors

Wrapped separately but also in the kidney dish are suturing instruments:

1 stitch scissors
1 small needle holder (This is a personal preference; some midwives may prefer a large needle holder.)
1 dissecting forceps, toothed or untoothed
1 small Spencer Wells forceps
To the right of the kidney dish there is a little metal box inside which is **Syntometrine 1 ml** and **ergometrine 0.5 mgm,** a **2 ml syringe, 2 needles** and a **spirit injection swab.**
To the left there is a **mucus extractor.**
These items are placed like this so that if on arrival at a home the birth is imminent the bag can be opened and the essentials are immediately to hand. In the bag there is also:

Obstetric cream
A supply of sterile plastic gloves

In a paper bag marked BABY
  2 cord clamps

Another mucus extractor
Layrngoscope with neonatal blade or other resuscitation
equipment *with which you are familiar*, for example a
baby ambu-bag
2 Endotracheal tubes of different sizes
A fine gastric tube, litmus paper, a 10 ml syringe
2 × 2 ml syringes, 2 small needles
Baby drugs: **Konakion 1 mgm** and **neonatal naloxone 2 ml**
ampoules

A paper bag marked SUTURING, containing:
20 ml syringe and needle
Local anaesthetic 0.5% or 1% lignocaine
2/0 catgut on a small round-bodied needle for posterior
vaginal wall
0 catgut on a tapercut needle for muscle
Black silk for skin sutures

There is considerable variation of opinion about the 'best'
materials to use for perineal suturing. Various studies have
been done to compare the long- and short-term advantages
of different materials and types of repairs. Community midwives are at an advantage in that we will usually be giving the
postnatal care to the women whose perinea we have sutured
and we rapidly learn which way we do best.

Paper bag marked BLOODS containing:
2 small bottles with anticoagulant, one for cord blood, one
for maternal blood
1 plain bottle for maternal blood
5 ml syringe and needle for taking cord blood
20 ml syringe and **needle** and **tourniquet** for taking maternal
blood

Each community midwife should inform herself of the requirements in her particular area and laboratory.

Also in the bag:
2 urethral catheters. Catheterisation is always best avoided
but occasionally it is essential. We need to be always aware

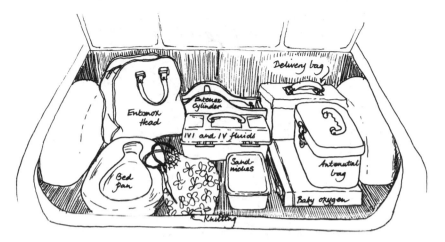

that each time we pass a catheter, even taking the most careful aseptic precautions, we are hazarding that woman's urinary tract. Many chronic urinary infections in women can be traced back to a catheterisation in childbirth. The midwife should ensure that she has good quality catheters, pliable but sufficiently firm to pass over a baby's head if catheterisation must be undertaken when the head is low in the pelvis.

1 amnihook

Glycerine suppositories

Phosphate disposable enema

These last two items one will use very rarely, particularly the enema, but occasionally one does find a woman whose rectum is absolutely full of hard faeces and who is greatly relieved by a gently given enema.

There are various **small basic dressing packs** that many midwives will wish to include in their bags.

Entonox equipment should be carried and regularly serviced. In cold weather it is very important that the cylinders of Entonox are not exposed to temperatures below 0°C (32°F). They should be stored at above 10°C (50°F). So don't be tempted to leave a cylinder in the boot of the car or the garage overnight in winter. If the cylinder has been exposed to low temperature the gases may have separated, and it is dangerous to use. It should be placed in warm water, about

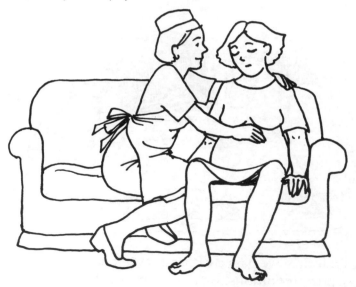

blood heat, for five minutes only, taking care not to get the valve wet, and then shaken and inverted several times to remix the gases.

Oxygen in small cylinders should be carried with a suitable apparatus for delivering it to a baby by face mask.

Many midwives also carry an **intravenous-giving set** and **intravenous fluids** such as Haemaccel (a synthetic form of plasma) or Hartmann's solution in case of postpartum haemorrhage. (Caroline and Mary have used theirs once each at a home birth.)

Most midwives will supply each woman with a large polythene bag containing **inco pads, sanitary pads** and a few vaginal examination packs which can be collected from the hospital. Individual midwives will identify their own needs in their own practices. A few fortunate midwives may still be able to supply the home confinement boxes.

CARE OF THE WOMAN IN LABOUR AT HOME

The requirements are the same as for good midwifery practice in hospital when caring for a normal woman in physiological labour: observe her condition, the condition of the fetus, the progress of the labour, and encourage, support, be tuned in to her needs and wishes, and keep contemporaneous records as required by our rules.

The various methods of pain relief as discussed in Chapter 5, with the exception of epidural anaesthesia, can all be used in the home. Midwives used to working in hospital are often amazed to see how much less chemical pain relief is used at home births, and how much variety there is in the ways that women alleviate the pain of labour. The woman in her own home, in control of what is happening, feels much more able to tell us when and if she needs the help of pain-relieving drugs.

The woman feels so much freer to move around. It is her kitchen, her bedroom, her living-room. We are the guests, and even in strong labour she will often still be undertaking her hostess role. Is that chair comfortable? Would we like some tea? (In this setting it is *we* who ask if we might use the lavatory.) There is so much more available to distract and relieve pain at home, things to lean on, things to do. If labour is long and she wants to curl up, she will do it in her own familiar bed or on her own sofa.

As the second stage approaches we will prepare for the birth, checking that we have the essentials laid out on our trays or surfaces and that the woman is getting herself into a position where she will be as comfortable as possible to give birth.

IT IS NOT NECESSARY TO TRY TO TURN A HOME INTO AN IMITATION OF A HOSPITAL DELIVERY ROOM. In the home babies emerge from their mother's bodies into their mother's arms gently and easily. The baby should be encouraged to suckle at the breast if that is the mother's wish. The midwife will manage the third stage, having regard to the wishes of the parents and according to her clinical judgement. Many women who elect to give birth at home will express a wish to avoid being given any drugs, and this may include the oxytocic drugs that are given at delivery to manage the third stage actively by controlled cord traction.

It is important to discuss this carefully with the woman

antenatally and, while respecting her wishes, we should describe the circumstances in which we feel that the administration of an oxytocic drug would be vital. Should the woman refuse categorically to have an oxytocic under any circumstances (and neither of us has ever had this happen) then the midwife should discuss the case with the supervisor of midwives, and write in the notes details of the discussion with the woman and with the supervisor.

After the third stage, it is a good idea to check the blood loss, the fundus, the baby, then clear the bed or delivery area as quickly as possible, to avoid damage to bedding, furnishings etc., and then leave the mother comfortable with her partner or friends to enjoy getting to know the baby. We can go off to have a careful look at the placenta and membranes, usually in the bathroom or kitchen, take cord blood if necessary and write up our notes, register and the birth notification. Some women may want to examine the placenta with us and we should ask about this before we remove it.

Should the perineum require suturing this can be done either immediately, or in the absence of bleeding from the perineum it can be left for a little while if the mother wishes. If there is just a little 'nick' of the fourchette or skin that only requires one or two stitches they can be inserted very quickly often before the placenta is delivered, and without the need for local anaesthetic. Some midwives find this is particularly easy if the woman has given birth in the left lateral position, but it can be done in the all fours or semi-dorsal position.

If there has been a second degree tear or an episiotomy has been necessary, the lithotomy position or something like it is desirable. How does one achieve this in the home?

The woman can be assisted to lie across her bed with her buttocks just at the edge and her feet on two chairs. The midwife either sits on a chair between her legs or kneels on a soft cushion. Spread an inco pad on the floor and put the bucket for spills and rubbish on the inco pad. Get your assistant to hold the light or position the anglepoise, put the necessary instruments and pack on a chair, and off you go, observing the same technique that you would use in hospital.

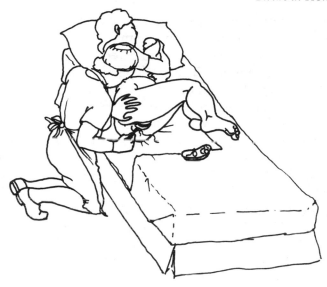

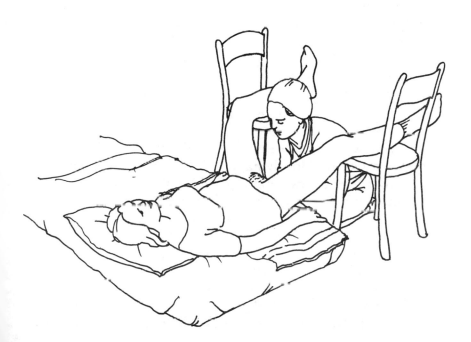

While it is no longer specified in the midwives' rules how long we should remain with the woman, most midwives will remain for a *minimum* of one hour after delivery, many of us remain for much longer. It must depend on the condition of the individual mother and baby.

We should help the mother to have a bath or a bed bath and generally freshen up. She should have passed urine and her fundus should be firm and central, the lochia should be normal. Demonstrate to the mother and another responsible adult in the house what the contracted uterus feels like. A firm ball like grapefruit in your tummy, and then show them how a contraction can be rubbed up, and say that if they feel too much blood is being lost and the bleeding is not stopping they should rub the tummy as we have shown them until they can feel the hard ball. This is so easy to do and it is such a simple precaution to take before one leaves the house.

The baby may be bathed or washed. If there is a great deal of vernix, it may be gently removed with almond oil. If vernix is left in the axillae it can occasionally cause a soreness. We will check the baby just as we would do in the hospital and write our findings in the notes. It is sensible to show the mother and another person how to lie the baby on its side head-down to assist mucus to drain and to mention that if the baby seems spluttery and mucosy, that it is capable of clearing its own airway, but holding it as shown will assist the process.

Having written up the notes we leave the house, probably tired but with that lovely happy 'high' and sense of achievement that reminds us what a privilege it is to be a midwife. We shouldn't be so euphoric that we forget to tell them exactly how they can get in touch with us, should there be any concern about the condition of mother or baby.

At the first available opportunity the midwife should clean, restock and check her bag and equipment. This is vital. Slumping into bed at 2 a.m. without having restocked your bag guarantees being called at 3 a.m. to someone in labour.

During the day, a return visit should be made within four

hours but few parents will thank us for a visit in the early hours. If the birth has taken place after 9 p.m. the family should be first visit on the list in the morning.

The community midwife attending home births may be working alone. She may be working with another midwife, with a student midwife or with a medical practitioner who may be the woman's usual general practitioner, or another doctor with whom she has contracted for maternity care. Most community midwives will know the general practitioners in their area and will have established relationships with them.

While it is perfectly acceptable for a midwife to attend a case on her own responsibility as a practising midwife, many women like their doctor to be involved and it can enhance the doctor's relationship with the family if she/he is around at the time of the birth. The matter of how and when the doctor is involved should ideally be a flexible affair, discussed by the woman, her midwife and doctor. Sometimes the doctor will visit during labour, sometimes be present at the birth to support and help. Often the doctor will call after the birth to admire and welcome the new patient to the practice and make a neonatal examination of the baby. As community midwives we should seek to work with our medical colleagues in a relationship of mutual respect for each other's roles as practising midwife and medical practitioner to the family.

Most planned home births take place normally and easily at home but there is about a 10% shift in planned place of delivery from home to hospital. Some of this alteration of plan will take place in the antenatal period as complications of pregnancy occur which will indicate the need for the birth to take place in hospital. Sometimes changes in the woman's social circumstances will mean a change in plan. Occasionally conditions will arise during the labour that will indicate the need to transfer to hospital. This is not 'things going wrong' but 'this woman in this labour needs help'. We should try to anticipate this need for help and transfer before there is a situation of something 'going wrong'.

The following indications for transfer to hospital are not exhaustive but are given as a general guide.

- The labour, having become established, is failing to progress. This is not just a matter of the latent or resting periods that can occur in normal labours, but is a labour that is outside the normal pattern of ongoing progress, where the presenting part fails to descend and advance, and the cervix fails to efface and dilate.
- A woman whose labour is causing her great pain, possibly with an occipito-posterior position, when she may need the help of epidural anaesthesia and transfer should be considered.
- A malposition or malpresentation of the baby becoming apparent during labour: face presentation, brow presentation.
- Failure of the presenting part to advance during the second stage. Should this happen the midwife should critically re-examine her management during the first stage to see if there were any indications of potential difficulties that were missed. Transfer during the second stage can be very traumatic for the woman, and very often in retrospect we can see where the difficulty in second stage could have been predicted and an earlier transfer arranged. Working in groups and discussing with other midwives is invaluable on these occasions in seeking to improve one's practice.
- Heavy bleeding during the third stage, or retained placenta causing a deterioration in the mother's condition, requires transfer to hospital by the emergency obstetric service.

The last circumstance is the emergency that many midwives commencing work in the community fear most. The dangers of postpartum haemorrhage are commonly cited by those opposed to home births. It was an emergency that was not uncommon in the days when most births occurred at home. In those days, we must remember, women were often malnourished, of high parity, modern oxytocic drugs were not available and operative deliveries were performed at home. It is important to get this undoubted emergency in perspective. It is extremely rare that following a normal, non-interventional first and second stage of labour, that the uterus, having functioned efficiently, ceases to do so in the third stage. In this extremely rare event the midwife will administer an oxytocic (ergometrine 0.5 or Syntometrine 1 ml) by intramuscular or intravenous injection, and send for the most appropriate medical aid. Under normal circumstances this will be the emergency obstetric service. If the midwife carries an IV set and has been trained in its use an intravenous infusion can be commenced. The midwife must ensure that the woman's bladder is empty and if necessary should catheterise her. The midwife can also rub the uterus to stimulate contractions, and encourage the baby to suckle.

In the absence of bleeding and with a mother in good condition a delay in the third stage can often be overcome by vigilant patience. If we have used Syntometrine the cervix may have clamped down before the placenta has passed through it. Wait patiently, observing the mother, recording her pulse and blood pressure frequently. Usually within an hour the cervix will relax and out will come the placenta. During a physiological third stage there can be quite a considerable latent period. The uterus has contracted and retracted, there is no bleeding, but the placenta is *in situ*. Patience is required. The baby can be encouraged to suckle and then the mother will feel a contraction and the placenta will emerge. Blowing into a bottle can aid the expulsion of the placenta and so can the assistance of gravity, either by sitting the woman on a large comfortable bed pan or by getting her to stand up.

Should these measures fail and the placenta still not emerge the midwife needs to consider the possibility of an abnormally adherent placenta and the need to transfer so it can be removed manually. Medical aid should be sought, this will be either the medical practitioner booked for the case or the registrar at the local maternity unit. Transfer in our view

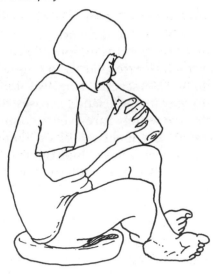

should *always* be by ambulance with an intravenous drip *in situ*. The midwife and registrar should discuss whether transfer should be by the obstetric emergency service or by ordinary ambulance. There is no immediate emergency if the woman's condition is good and there has been no excessive bleeding, but in the circumstances of a retained placenta this can change quite quickly. During the journey the placenta could partially detach and bleeding could ensue. Local circumstances, such as distances to be travelled and any likely delays, should be taken into account.

The question one asks oneself is how long should one wait with a placenta *in situ* before transfer? There can be no hard and fast rules, each case must be considered on its merits and the geography and other local factors assessed. But a delay of over one and a half hours, even in the absence of bleeding and with the woman in good condition, should indicate a need to transfer. Many midwives would consider that one hour is a sufficient time to wait before transfer.

During a labour the need to transfer to hospital may be indicated by a deterioration in the fetal condition signified by any irregularity or slowing of the fetal heart. With a portable heart monitor the fetal heart can be listened to during and for thirty seconds after a contraction. What would show on a monitor as 'dips' will be immediately apparent. Without a fetal heart monitor but with experience one can listen just as well with a Pinard's stethoscope. There is no need to lie the mother down. If the Pinard's is positioned and then the bell of a binaural stethoscope is put over the ear hole of the Pinard's one can listen comfortably.

Meconium staining of the liquor during the first stage may indicate a need to transfer. If the membranes rupture at the onset of the second stage and meconium is present there may be no time to transfer particularly if the mother is multiparous. In our view the best way to deliver the baby in these circumstances is with the mother on all fours. In an occipito-anterior position the head will be born facing the midwife, who can then suck out the mouth and nasopharynx while the chest is still compressed by the birth canal. If there is thick meconium sucked out it is wise to transfer the case to hospital, because even if the baby initially appears in good condition, if meconium has been inspired, the baby's condition can deteriorate rapidly and need urgent intensive care.

The new community midwife undertaking births at home often has a considerable amount of conditioning to overcome about the safety aspect of home births. Apart from the postpartum haemorrhage fear already discussed, the other 'what if' commonly mentioned is: 'What if there is a "flat" baby?' Again this is a perfectly reasonable fear for a midwife accustomed to working in a hospital surrounded by sophisticated resuscitation equipment, but again it is important to get the problem into perspective. Yes, babies are sometimes born in poor condition, but these are not usually babies born at home to healthy women following normal pregnancies and easy births. Vigilance and transfer to hospital care when appropriate will mean that very few babies are born in poor condition at home. Having said that, no system and no midwife is perfect, and there will be the baby who does need active resuscitation at home. The midwife should ensure that she is equipped for this unlikely event, by checking her equipment: laryngoscope, endotracheal tubes, oxygen, baby ambu bag. It is also our duty to ensure that we maintain our skills. Every six months or so go into the hospital and practise on the plastic doll kept in most labour wards for the purpose, either supervised by one of the paediatric consultants or by one of the skilled and experienced staff of the Special Care Baby Unit. This is something that could be discussed and arranged by one's supervisor of midwives. Opportunities to learn and practise these skills are often available at the excellent study days organised in various parts of the country by midwives' organisations.

This chapter on birth at home has ended by detailing the problems that can arise. We need to remember that for the normal healthy woman a booking for birth at home is a matter of choice and there is no evidence to suggest that birth at home is any less physically safe than in hospital for mother or baby. There is some considerable evidence that for many women it is a more positive and less traumatic and happier life event. Rona Campbell and Alison Macfarlane discuss this in detail in their well researched publication *Where to be Born: The Debate and the Evidence* (obtainable from the National Perinatal Epidemiology Unit, Oxford).

It concerns us that when we book a woman for a home birth we are expected to list to her all the dangers of having a baby at home, so that we are sure that her decision is a result of informed choice. However, when a woman books into a hospital for a hospital birth is she ever given a list of the dangers of hospital birth? Or even the dangers of hospital birth in that particular unit? Imagine her being told: 'We think we ought to tell you that in this unit we have a particularly resistant staphylococcus which crops up from time to time, and we have a consultant obstetrician whose caesarean rate is twice the national average and you are booked under him. Also the epidural team is having problems getting its quota of epidurals practised by their learners, so that every woman here is under great pressure to have an epidural and our percentage is running at 65% of women having epidurals this month.'

It makes you think.

Reference

Campbell, Rona, MacFarlane, Alison. (1987). *Where to be Born: The Debate and the Evidence*. Oxford: National Perinatal Epidemiology Unit.

Chapter Five

The Relief of Pain in Labour

As midwives working in the community both of us deliver babies at home and in hospital. Between us we looked after 64 woman in 1987, 29 at home and 35 in hospital.

One of us, on looking through old registers, discovered that in the 1950s and 60s, when practically all the women delivered at home, much more pethidine and Trilene (which was the inhalational analgesia in use at the time) was used now when we care for more of our women in hospitals.

We discussed what has led to the use of less analgesia and what has changed over the years. We realised that the greatest change has occurred in the women themselves. Antenatal classes as we know them now did not exist in the 1950s and 60s. Women today are much better informed, and much less inhibited and afraid, than the women of 25 years ago. Pain thresholds are increased when women know what is happening to them, and within them. Fathers are much more involved and supportive now. A man who was with his wife was unusual in the 50s. Now it's the other way round and the man who is not there is unusual. Men have learnt to be more sensitive, and expect to be more supportive to women in labour.

The other great change that we discussed, was in us, the midwives. We both feel that we have learnt to listen to, and to respond to a woman's needs in sharing her care with her. As we have watched and learnt just how emotionally and physically strong women can be in childbirth, we have learnt to be much more 'with' women. Since the time that Grantly Dick Read pointed out the fear-tension-pain cycle, midwives have had a much better understanding of how we can at least avoid increasing the pain of labour. We are not so naive to suggest that alleviating fear eliminates tension and pain, but it certainly helps. So the reduction of fear is the first thing we should be doing when we are considering the management of pain in labour. This starts at the very first meeting when we begin to get to know each other and continues right through her pregnancy as a friendship develops.

The ways we help to relieve pain can be thought of as a collection of tools and the art of 'pain relief' is selecting, with the woman, the right tool, or combination of tools for her particular labour.

Our first tool is ourselves, our physical presence, the reassurance that we bring, that we know that this process works, that we are not frightened by labour, though we respect its power. That we know the end result will be a lovely healthy baby, and that the woman can do it. We need to recognise when to be strong, quiet and patient. We need to be able to sit quietly. If this is difficult, knitting may help, or a book or crochet. Our physical presence need not necessarily be within the room if it is a home birth, sometimes it is nice for the woman if we sit outside the room, or downstairs in the sitting room so that she and her partner have some privacy, but she needs to know that we are only a groan away and that the moment she wants us we will be there like a shot.

This is unlike the situation in many hospitals when the woman will need us there all the time, our familiar sounds and presence make the room more normal and familiar and we act as a buffer when strangers enter, and act as a defence against invasion.

Our next tool is our voices: soothing, encouraging, crooning, strengthening, but tempered to the needs of each individual woman: 'You can do it Joyce, the baby's nearly here.' 'Well done, Jane that was wonderful.' 'Becky you are managing so well you are superwoman.' 'Not long now Rene, not long, nearly there, soon be over. You coped beautifully with that contraction. You are magnificent.' 'Each pain is one less, each contraction is one nearer to saying Happy Birthday.'

Sometimes distraction helps. 'Could you pop along to the loo after the next contraction, Jean? I'd like you to empty your bladder.' 'Look at this mobile/blind cord/my nose, concentrate on it.' 'Count the squares in the ceiling and see how many you get to during each contraction.' Often, though, the best way to use our voices is to stay silent, sitting quietly and contentedly, and sometimes shushing others who are trying to talk. 'Ssh, she wants quiet to concentrate.' 'Ssh, talking distracts her, she just needs to know we are here, she doesn't want to hear our voices.'

Our hands are important tools, touching a woman, patting her, stroking her, but always remembering that some women do not like to be touched. Back rubbing gently or firmly, in time with a woman's breathing; 'butterfly' stroking across her abdomen; deep massaging of her shoulders if they get tense; deep massaging of her friend's/partner's/mum's shoulders if they get stiff; just a hand on her arm to say, 'I'm here, you're doing fine.'

Another tool is heat and cold. Hot water bottles over the lower abdomen or the lower back are marvellous for some women, hot flannels to the perineum are immensely comforting in second stage especially for primigravid women or where the perineum is scarred. Bathing in warm water can be a huge comfort – relaxing both for the woman and her cervix. Bathing can also be a distraction to the pain and help her to melt into her contractions.

Cold is also useful, as was discovered during a cold winter when an apology was given for freezing cold hands as a woman's back was rubbed, but the woman thought they felt lovely so a hot water bottle filled with iced water was used very effectively throughout the first stage. Flannels or sanitary pads wrung out with iced water give great relief in the second stage if haemorrhoids are prolapsing, held firmly over the anus they are a great help.

Mobility is a very useful tool. Many women like to be mobile and move around in labour, some like to curl up and rest. Some women need physical support, another body to learn against during a contraction, a hand to squeeze when the going is tough, a pair of shoulders to help them along to the lavatory. Often it seems that our hospital facilities are only planned to deliver babies, but do not provide facilities to

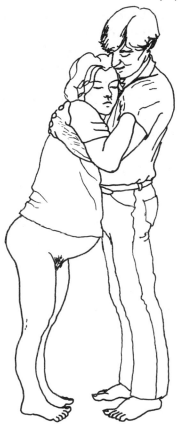

encourage women to give birth. At home there are chairs, sofas, tables, worktops over which women can lean, moving around as they feel the need.

Many women who are able to melt into their contractions, who can relax totally, perhaps aided by dim lighting, reduction in stimuli, learned rhythmic breathing patterns, warm deep baths, or repeating mantras, release their own endorphins, the pain-relieving substances which the body can produce. These women who have received no drugs may appear 'drugged' by the end of a labour. It is important that the midwife does not confuse this with fatigue and exhaustion. The exhausted woman will have a fast pulse and her contractions may diminish in strength and frequency, the woman producing endorphins will have a pulse within the normal range and her uterus will be contracting efficiently.

The next tool is assessment of progress, explaining and sharing with the woman. If she is dilating slowly and labour is likely to be long we should be thinking about tiredness, and depending upon time of day, it is often worth tucking a woman in early labour into bed with a couple of dichloralphenazone tablets and a hot drink in the hope of getting some sleep. This is where going to the home of a woman who thinks she might be in labour to assess her is so useful, as borne out by Klein *et al.*'s study discussed in Chapter 3 (page 41), which showed that when women were assessed at home in early labour, they went into hospital further advanced in labour, and the need for analgesia and instrumental deliveries was much reduced as compared with women going into hospital to be assessed in early labour. This is why it is important for any scheme which aims to provide compassionate and supportive care of women in labour, that the midwife should be able to visit the woman at home and assess her labour and advise her from there. The midwife can go to a woman's home in early labour, sit with her for a bit, examine her, reassure her, and tuck her up in bed. Most of us are far more likely to rest in our own beds with our own partners beside us than anywhere else, though we mustn't forget that a few women will feel more secure and have less fear in hospital, especially if there are over-anxious family members around at home.

An extremely important tool is our ears: to listen to women, not just to their words but to the noises they make. Many women have been conditioned to be so stiff upper-lipped that making a lot of noise in labour is seen as unacceptable, and many women who have made only the gentlest of noises during a long and gruelling labour apologise profusely. The other problem we have to face and overcome when being with women who are making a noise is to resist the temptation to *do* something for them. For many women, yelling, moaning, groaning, keening or screaming helps to relieve pain. Sometimes a woman starts to make a noise, becomes inhibited and controls herself. When that happens we both try to say 'Does it help to yell?' and encourage her to make as much noise as she needs. It can be helpful to talk about it antenatally. Tell her she might also hear another woman making a noise, but not to think she is in agony – she may well be relieving her pain by making that noise. Sometimes women seem to find relief in yelling just when they have an anterior lip of cervix. It may be there is an association between a stiff upper-lip and a persistent stiff anterior lip! But we mustn't forget women who are in fact crying for help and who may need help from the next group of tools we discuss.

Our next tools are the pharmacological ones we have access to. Pethidine can be an immensely useful drug, despite the well known side effects, the danger of depression of the baby's respiratory centre and the disadvantage of sometimes making the baby sleepy for a few days after the birth. But it can be absolutely wonderful for the mother whose contractions are strong and painful, particularly if on vaginal examination the cervix feels tight and tense. It seems that this often happens in primigravidae at around 6 cm dilatation. We use small doses (50 mg). Usually this is enough for the woman to have a short refreshing snooze and to carry on with her labour. More can always be given but if women are knocked out with 150 + mg they may become unable to push in the second stage.

The secret of the successful use of Entonox is the timing of its administration. Sitting with women, timing their contractions, it becomes apparent that the time lag between commencing Entonox inhalation and obtaining benefit varies from woman to woman from 10 to 25 seconds, usually occurring around 15 seconds. The importance of starting to take the Entonox just as a contraction starts cannot be over emphasised. Sometimes the midwife can pick up the start of the contraction with her hand on the abdomen before the woman feels it. A monitor can be useful in this connection too. The end of the first stage is when many women find Entonox most useful. It can also be used during the second stage if the woman wishes, though once the second stage is established, and the woman is pushing, she will often discard the Entonox and comment that the pain is less though the effort is enormous.

Epidurals are immensely useful, the need for them is rare but they can be of enormous benefit in the following cases, where a community midwife could be in attendance:

- The woman who has transferred to hospital care due to pre-eclampsia and where induction of labour is indicated. The epidural, in addition to providing excellent pain relief in an induced labour, which is often much more severe than a spontaneous labour, will also have a desirable hypotensive effect.
- The long painful labour where one transfers to hospital care and the labour is augmented with an oxytocic. This is frequently associated with a posterior position of the vertex.

Community midwives, because their main work is in the field of normal physiological labours, may have little opportunity to become proficient or experienced in the management of labouring women under epidural. If in attendance in hospital with a woman requiring epidural anaesthesia it is important to be quite frank with the labour ward staff. Most labour ward staff are only too pleased to help, teach, and guide their community colleagues who ask for help. This is where the good relationships between community and hospital staff, as discussed in Chapter 13, are so important.

An epidural which works perfectly – and the anaesthetist should always be recalled if it doesn't – can enable a woman to have a positive happy experience of birth, which could otherwise have been an exhausting nightmare. Epidurals are wonderful when used to relieve women's distress. They are not so useful when used to relieve that other condition which can occur and which could be the subject of another book – midwives' and obstetricians' distress.

To conclude, the relief of pain in labour is an enormously important part of midwife's care. We have attempted to discuss it as broadly as possible. Every woman's pain is different, and while we now have the technology, maybe we need to develop the sensitivity to respond appropriately to each and every woman's individual need – whether it be for a back rub, a change of position, or an epidural.

References

Dick Read, Grantly. (1956). *Childbirth Without Fear*. London: William Heinemann Medical Books.

Klein, N., Lloyd, I., Redman, C., Bull M., Turnbull, A. C. (1983). A comparison of low-risk pregnant women booked for delivery in two systems of care: shared care (consultant) and integrated general practice unit. *British Journal of Obstetrics and Gynaecology*; **90**: 118–28 (February).

Melzack, R. (1973). *The Puzzle of Pain*. Harmondsworth: Penguin Books.

Melzack, R., Wall, P. D. (1965). Pain mechanisms, a new theory. *Science*; **150** (3699): 971–9.

Sosa, R., Kennel, J., Klaus, M., Robertson, S., Urrutia, J. (1980) The effect of a supportive companion on perinatal problems, length of labour, and mother–infant interaction. *New England Journal of Medicine*; **303**: 597–600.

Chapter Six

The Community Midwife and Postnatal Care

'NOW, WHAT SHALL I DO WITH IT?'

The essence of postnatal care is to produce a woman who is confident in her ability to care for and nurture her child. Our involvement is so short and so limited, that we should at all times be building up the woman's, and her partner's, confidence in their own abilities, so that when we slip away on Day 10 or Day 14, 21 or 28, we know that these parents are competent and confident and that this child is safe and cared for.

We can do this by helping them to realise how much the baby likes them, how much the baby gazes at them and listens to their voices. The gratifying aspect of young children (especially from about 3 months onwards) is that they love their parents unconditionally – that the parents don't have someone who is critical of them but someone who thinks that they are the most wonderful thing that has ever come into his life, a small fan club! It isn't until parents have grown up considerably and have teenaged children that they are criticised and viewed with judgmental eyes.

The other confidence booster for new parents is to acknowledge how well the parents carry out practical tasks on their baby.

- 'You have got the nappy on neatly, John.'
- 'She does like you bathing her, doesn't she?'
- 'He looks really comfortable when you feed him like that.'

It is important for us to voice these encouragements, and this is not easy for us as a profession because so much feedback that midwives receive is negative –

- 'No, that's not how you should do it.'

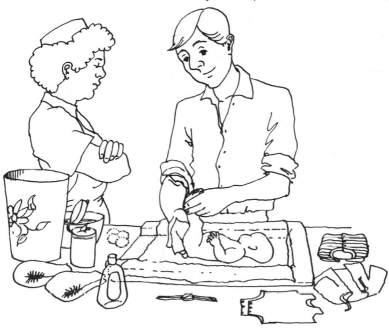

- 'Please come and see me in my office over Mrs Brown's labour.'

so that they themselves are not used to positive feedback. How much more helpful to be told:

- 'When you conduct a delivery it's so beautifully peaceful, no fuss or panic.'
- 'Can I watch you stitching? I'm told that you are so good at it.'
- 'Mrs Brown told me that she couldn't have done without you during her labour, she says you were so supportive and gave her strength.'

Positive feedback enables our confidence to grow, it makes us feel good and it allows us to progress. New parents need it more than most. Their whole world has been turned upside down, they are not getting sufficient sleep, they are tired, overwhelmed and trying to find a way to bring up this baby, stop this baby crying, find a few minutes in order to have a bath. Some women feel that they are going mad because they have so little control over their lives and a few well-chosen phrases acknowledging what she is doing with her baby can work wonders for her self-confidence. Postnatal care does not vary very much whether it is happening at home or in hospital but different aspects of it are apparent in the different environments.

POSTNATAL VISIT AT HOME

The Midwives' Rules include the statement that the postnatal period is 'a period of not less than ten and not more than twenty-eight days after the end of labour, during which the continued attendance of a midwife on a mother is requisite.' The Midwives' Code of Practice quotes the European Community Midwives' Directive 80/155/EEC Article 4, which says (relating to postnatal care): 'Member states shall ensure that midwives are at least entitled to take up and pursue the following activities ... to care for and monitor the progress of the mother in the postnatal period and to give all necessary advice to the mother on infant care to enable her to ensure the optimum progress of the newborn infant.'

Most midwives take this to mean that they will visit the new mother and baby twice a day for the first three days, and then daily for the next seven days. After 10 days the midwife uses her discretion and visits perhaps every four to five days until the child is four weeks old.

It is usual to check the mother first if possible because after you have disturbed the baby she/he may well be crying and needing to suckle, and once the baby is fixed you can leave. If the baby is checked first the baby is crying the whole time the mother is being checked and this will upset her and put her on edge.

POSTNATAL EXAMINATION OF THE MOTHER

'How are you feeling?' – and the midwife sits down to listen as if she has all the time in the world. The woman needs to tell someone how she is and how motherhood is affecting

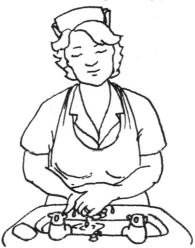

her. She has a great need to talk through her labour, even if you are the midwife who was with her throughout it – she will need to talk through every minute of the birth several times so that she can assimilate it. If you do not have the time for incorporating this into your postnatal visits, you need to do something about your workload (see Chapter 11).

If you are the midwife who delivered this woman it is incredibly useful for you to know what your actions meant to the woman and how she perceived the labour and birth.

As the midwife listens to the mother she is all the time observing the woman and assessing her emotional and physical condition and interpreting her body language. The midwife then washes her hands and performs a physical examination of the mother and then the baby. Temperature, pulse and blood pressure should be recorded but none of these are necessarily done daily or ritualistically. Do them as and when you consider they are appropriate. Some midwives say that if a woman is feverish they know anyway and that it is ridiculous to take her temperature, a hand on her forehead is enough. The great advantage of taking the woman's temperature is that she feels that you are actually checking her physical condition and this is heartening for her, and the other advantage is that you can write in the notes Temperature 98.4°F or Temp. 37°C, Pulse 84 and Blood pressure 120/70.

A woman's pulse is probably the most important indicator of her well-being. If it is rapid and thready has she an infection? Or perhaps she is bleeding? Or anaemic? If the pulse is strong and regular usually the woman is healthy.

While observing the woman the midwife will have noted pallor, normal colour or flushed. Check breasts – whether they are soft, comfortable, lactating, engorged, whether her nipples are sore, cracked, inverted and ask how she feels breastfeeding is progressing.

If you feel that brassieres are important, advice can be given at this stage. It is not essential actually to gaze at the woman's breasts each day – the woman is capable of telling you how they feel. But often women produce their breasts the minute you ask how they are. This may be a comfortable reaction to your questions, but it could be an indication that the woman now feels that her body is somehow 'public property' and can indicate the damage done to her self-image by the way she has been treated during childbirth.

The first indicator of breast problems can be a flushed triangle in one of the quadrants of the breast. In order to encourage circulation in the breast and to speed up the emptying of that portion of the breast, the baby should be fed in different positions. Try the 'rugger tackle' hold with the baby's body under the mother's arm, or with the mother lying on her side and the baby suckling.

If the woman complains of sore nipples then it is important to watch her feeding her baby in order to ascertain that the baby is fixed on well, that the nipple and areola are well back in the baby's mouth so that the mother's nipple is pressed against the baby's soft palate and is not being rubbed by the baby's tongue every time she/he sucks. Very sore nipples are almost invariably a result of poor positioning. Another cause of very tender nipples is the rare occasion when a baby has oral thrush and the mother has thrush on her nipples.

The woman needs to empty her bladder so that her fundus

can be palpated. Is it central, firm, well contracted, involuting? Some units use a tape measure and the fundus is measured daily. Other midwives just ascertain the progress of the fundus compared to how it was the day before. The other aspect of palpating the fundus which is important is whether or not it is tender. If it is tender when touched – either uterine infection (puerperal fever), or the retention of some placental tissue in the uterus, in which case a secondary postpartum haemorrhage could be a possibility. The pulse needs to be checked. In the case of retained products, it will be faster than normal. Often after-pains will have persisted longer than the usual 48 hours as the uterus tries to expel the retained products. The administration of ergometrine tablets, 0.5 mg three times a day for three days, can help the uterus to expel the retained products. The woman needs to be told to expect the passage of a clot, increased after-pains and what to do should she begin to bleed heavily (immediately contact the GP or the midwife and be prepared for hospital admission). The use of ergometrine is not universally favoured and there are mixed views on its efficacy, but a drug which has been used by midwives since Old Testament times could be said to have withstood the test of time! If the midwife needs to give ergometrine she needs to alert the GP, in case the woman needs to be transferred to hospital for an 'evacuation of retained products of conception'. What is happening is a deviation from normality and she is obliged to inform a doctor in such a situation.

Many women who have had babies before experience strong after-pains and need to be treated sympathetically because these can be extremely painful. Paracetamol can help, as can a hot water bottle or hot bath. Sympathy and reassurance that they should subside after 48 hours will help the mother to get through.

If the lochia smells offensive (and it has to be borne in mind that stale blood smells a bit 'fishy'), and the woman's fundus is tender, not involuting but feeling broad and 'boggy', it is important to deal with this urgently because of the danger of postpartum haemorrhage.

- The midwife can start the woman on a course of ergometrine tablets (500 mcgm–0.5 mg three times a day for three days).
- The woman must drink extra fluids, water, squash, tea, soup etc.
- A doctor needs to be informed. She/he may prescribe antibiotics and may discuss possible admission to hospital for an evacuation of retained products of conception.

Usually the fundus involutes steadily and the lochia smells of normal stale blood. The lochia needs to be examined to check on (a) smell; (b) colour. The normal progression is red, pink, brown, white but often the lochia is a mixture of two, e.g. pink/brown and can be quite watery. Often the lochia reverts a stage once the woman gets up and is doing more. It can become redder once she is going up and down stairs or taking her children to school even though the fundus is not palpable. If a couple have sexual intercourse this also makes the lochia flow red again.

The amount of lochia also needs to be recorded – profuse (be vigilant), normal, or scant flow. If the flow is scant and the fundus is not involuting, there may be a clot in the uterus. Warn the mother that this may come out soon and/or give her a course of ergometrine tablets.

Even when the woman's perineum is intact it needs to be examined to see whether the skin looks healthy and is healing well. Encouraging words are very important here – women are very afraid of the damage which has been inflicted on their perineum. It is wise to check that they are cleaning it well. Often a woman will be afraid to touch the area, particularly if she has had stitches or if she has haemorrhoids. It can be useful to accompany her to the bath and to encourage her to make a soapy lather on her hand and then to massage her perineum with that. This helps her to touch herself again and the massaging encourages circulation and so promotes healing.

It is important to encourage the woman to tighten her pelvic floor muscles and to give her feedback when you see the muscles actually moving. This will encourage her to do more exercises and will also stimulate blood circulation and aid healing.

If the woman has piles it might be helpful to her if you reduce them with a gloved finger and KY jelly. They may be too tender for that to be possible but they may benefit from the application of an icepack – a quarter pound packet of frozen peas is ideal for this as they are small and mould to the shape of the woman. If they are put in a clean polythene bag each time they are used, the colour from the packet will not mark the woman and the packet can be refrozen for her use again.

A clove of garlic inserted into the anus apparently reduces piles.

The other great boon for the woman is glycerine suppositories, especially if she is very fearful of having her bowels open, afraid that her stitches may burst, that her piles will come down, that her insides will fall out. If the midwife inserts two glycerine suppositories and tells the woman that they are made of jelly and will melt inside her and her faeces will slide out, many woman cannot wait the prescribed twenty minutes and rush to the lavatory within minutes, to come out beaming with the news that they 'have been'.

The words we use for describing the perineal area are of paramount importance; the woman's image of herself can be damaged permanently by our words if they are ill-chosen. For example, Andrea, the mother of a six-month-old baby, said: 'I'm like a barge down there, I daren't let my husband near me, I know he'll leave me when he knows that my pelvic floor muscles have completely gone.' When I asked her why she thought her perineum was in such an unlikely condition she described a midwife gazing at her pelvic floor in horror and saying, 'It's really gaping.' The midwife commenting on Andrea's sutured episiotomy had destroyed that woman's self-confidence with her ill-chosen words. Our words are very powerful. They are remembered, discussed, embroidered and assume enormous significance during this very sensitive time. We have to be very careful of what words we use, and to be positive and encouraging:

- 'You are doing your pelvic floor exercises well, I can see them working – well done, keep doing them during the day.'
- 'Your stitches are nice and clean, your skin looks healthy. It is healing well.'
- 'Your episiotomy is healing but it is slow, make sure that you massage it well with a soapy hand and keep exercising your pelvic floor muscles to get the blood circulating. Then it will be as good, if not better, than it was before you had your baby.'
- 'You look as if you've never had a baby down here.'
- 'Yes, you are right, you have got a little lump left where the stitches were, it will eventually get smaller and you could try and massage it with oil to help it on its way. Most women are aware of a change in their vulval area though no-one else would be able to tell. Anyone seeing you there for the first time wouldn't think anything of it, they would just think that that is how you are made.'
- 'Tighten your pelvic floor muscles for me – well done, they are strong'.

Suggestions for healing a perineum which is slow to heal are (all unevaluated):

- Pelvic floor exercises
- Lying on the front (to enable the two halves of the wound to go together)
- Washing every time the woman goes to the lavatory
- Using a hair dryer to dry the wound after washing and going to the lavatory
- Wearing no knickers to allow air to circulate
- Exposing the wound to the sunlight
- Treating any anaemia
- Good diet
- Calendula (a few drops) put in the bath water
- Calendula tincture on a sanitary towel

- Arnica 30 tablets (a homeopathic remedy): two tablets, four times a day following delivery for 3 to 4 days. Homeopathic remedies should not be touched with the hand but should be dropped underneath the tongue and absorbed. They should not be taken less than 20 minutes after eating or less than 20 minutes before eating. Coffee should not be drunk when taking homeopathic remedies and they take a very long time to be absorbed.
- Lotio rubra has been used for many years for promoting wound healing – a swab soaked in this and held against the stitches with a sanitary towel appears to aid healing and promote comfort.
- For tight scar tissue ultrasound administered by an obstetric physiotherapist seems to be beneficial.

When discussing contraception it is as well to warn women that they may not feel sexually aroused for many months after their baby is born. Many women are frightened of making love after having had stitches and for up to a year following childbirth many women experience vaginal dryness. Lovemaking can be made more comfortable by KY jelly. Following childbirth many women feel quite numb, and erotic arousal takes gentle and sensitive wooing by the woman's partner.

The woman needs to be asked about micturition and defecation. Women who have problems in passing urine after the birth of their baby can sometimes go if they are sitting in the bath, often when the plug has been pulled out. Other women find it easier to use a bedpan and to be lying down when they first try to pass urine, or in private in their own lavatory.

The woman's legs need to be checked for any signs of deep vein thrombosis – pain, tenderness, swelling, heat. It needs to be remembered that pulmonary embolism is the main cause of maternal mortality and it is invariably caused from a deep vein thrombosis in the leg. Women should not have pain in their legs after childbirth, they should be able to walk with ease – if they can't the reason needs to be investigated.

The woman needs to be shown postnatal exercises and

encouraged to do them. It is often a good idea to watch her doing them as you sip the cup of tea that, hopefully, you have been given! With you watching and encouraging her, she may be more likely to start doing them. Just offering her a chart with some exercises on may not be positive enough.

Many women have a gap in the *recti abdominis* muscles following delivery – if she is encouraged to feel it about once a week she will be able to notice that the gap becomes less and less as the weeks go by. A good exercise to alleviate this is for her to lie on the floor with her knees bent and arms behind her head: tightening her tummy muscles, she flattens her back against the floor and lifts her head and shoulders to the count of 10 – never lifting them so high that the tummy rises up in a point, only lifting as high as will allow her tummy to remain flat. She should do this up to 50 times a day, as well as practising good posture and pelvic tilts whilst standing.

CARE OF THE BABY

Especially if it is her first baby the mother will need help and encouragement in handling her baby.

One of the most essential skills she needs to acquire is how to change a nappy. At home it is useful to organise a 'nappy changing place' so that nappies can be changed quickly and smoothly. This place needs somewhere soft for the baby to lie on. It can be an old towel on a flat surface, or a nappy changing mat or a thick inco pad – or a chair in which the mother can sit comfortably and use her legs to form a good lap for the baby to lie in. The nappy changing place can also be on a flat surface, on top of a chest-of-drawers, on the floor, on a board over the bath, on a table.

In the nappy changing place there needs to be two or three clean nappies, a complete set of clean clothes for the baby, a towel, and something to clean the baby with – this can be water in a small bowl plus cotton wool or a baby sponge, baby wipes, baby lotion plus cotton wool, or baby oil plus cotton wool. Within easy access there needs to be a waste-

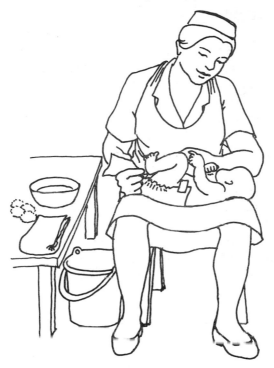

paper bin to receive rubbish and, if possible, a receptacle for dirty baby clothes.

Once the nappy changing place is organised, nappy changing is contained all in one place, can be performed quickly and efficiently and becomes much less of a chore. Some women have a nappy changing place on each floor if they live in a house; some have a portable one for going out, a bag with everything in it, which can also be transported around the house. This should be discussed antenatally and with the woman before she goes home from hospital.

The woman needs to be shown how to wash the baby's face and then his bottom – 'topping and tailing'. She also needs to know how to bath the baby, which can be done in all sorts of ways.

- It can be bathed with its Mum or Dad in the big bath. The feel of small firm naked skin against the parent's adult skin

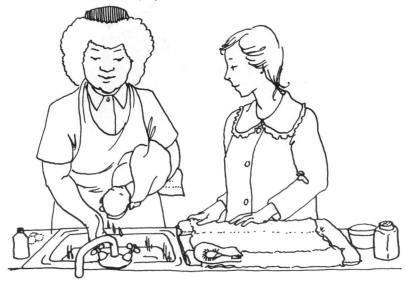

is glorious – the water should be comfortably warm for the adult to get into but not hot.

- The baby can be bathed in the sink as long as the taps don't drip or are covered with a flannel.
- The baby can be bathed in a washing-up bowl or even a plastic bucket.
- A baby bath is commonly used, but these are often very heavy to carry when they are full of water and the water tends to slop about.

The principles of bathing a baby are that the baby should end up clean and that it should have had its head kept above water. We write this because many amazing 'techniques' have been developed in the area of bathing a baby and the whole business has been made so frightening. There are now even special detergent-like substances to put in the baby's bath in order that parents needn't actively wash their children and can bypass the whole frightening technique. This seems tragic when one of the loveliest feelings is the feel of firm baby skin under your hand when you soap it and when this massage is a source of great pleasure for the baby. Soaping can be done outside the bath before putting the baby in the warm water or it can be done while the baby is lying in the bath supported by your other hand. Most people start at the top when washing a child and work down to the feet.

Before bathing a baby:

- The room should be warm, with doors and windows closed.
- Everything for the bath (cotton wool, soap, towel and wastepaper basket) should be ready.
- Everything for dressing the baby should be ready (nappy, cream or lotion, vest, bootees, babygro or nightdress, cardigan, shawl). The nappy should be left on until the last possible moment and the clean one put on again as soon as possible, for obvious reasons!

Bathing can take place in the evening to encourage the baby to sleep. It can also be done in the middle of the night if the baby is very fretful. Massage with almond oil can take place after the baby's bath as long as the room is well warmed.

POSTNATAL EXAMINATION OF THE BABY

The baby should be examined most days (but probably not on the day when he has been crying solidly for the past two hours and has just gone off to sleep).

The **baby's demeanour** is the most important indication of well-being, or lack of it:

- Is he alert and interested in life?
- Is he looking around enquiringly, aware of noises, listening when people talk directly at him?
- Is the baby's muscle tone good, and is he kicking and waving arms around? Or is the baby sleepy, lethargic, floppy?

The *baby's temperature* can be ascertained by touch and by being conscious of the temperature of the room the baby is in. An axillary temperature can be taken with a thermometer and, if absolutely necessary, a rectal temperature can be taken, but with awareness that this is an invasive procedure which can cause trauma to the rectal mucosa and can stimulate the parasympathetic nervous system and cause the baby to experience a degree of shock.

The *baby's eyes* should be clear and open. The eyelids may be swollen following delivery and there may be inflammation or pus inside them. If the eyes are sticky reassure the woman that this is not uncommon. It is often caused because the baby's tear ducts are not open fully yet. A solution of saline can be used to bathe the eyes – an eggcupful of water that has been boiled and has a few grains of salt added to it (about an eighth of a teaspoonful). Some midwives use sterile sachets of saline, some use weak cold tea or breast milk to bathe the baby's eyes. If the condition persists the GP needs to be informed so that she/he can prescribe antibiotic treatment.

The *baby's skin* – is it warm and smooth? Is it free of bruises, is there a rash or milk spots? Is it dry and flaky, peeling or cracked? Is there paronychia on any of the baby's fingers? Does the skin have the yellow tinge of physiological jaundice? If the baby is alert and suckling well the jaundice is not severe. The white light in the spectrum helps to speed the disappearance of the jaundice. You can intensify it by the use of white sheets in front of a window on a sunny day. The baby's eyes need to be protected from the glare and it is important to check that the baby is not becoming either too hot or too cold.

The *baby's mouth*. Is it clean and free of thrush, eagerly open when a breast or bottle approaches it?

The *umbilicus*. Is the cord clamp or ligature on securely? Has the cord clamp been removed? Is the cord drying up? Is the cord being treated with any potions or powders? Does the cord smell? (Not infrequent when blood has been trapped in it before clamping.) Is the cord on, hanging by a thread, off? Is the umbilicus dry, moist, clean, inflamed, purulent?

Is the baby *passing urine*? This can take up to five days to

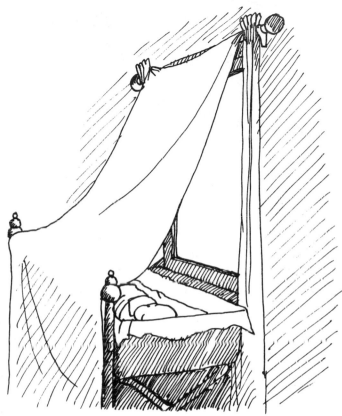

start, and if the baby doesn't pass urine for several days following delivery the first few urines may well have a pinkish colour because of the presence of salts (urates) in the urine.

Is the baby *passing stool*? Is it tarry black meconium, brown changing stool, yellow stool with flecks in which are reminiscent of cottage cheese, or do the baby's stools have a greenish tinge? Are the stools very liquid and explosive? This could be because the baby is feeding too quickly and if the mother attempts to feed the baby 'uphill' the flow will not be so rapid or more likely, that the baby is poorly positioned during breast feeding. Or you could enquire if the baby is being given drinks of water, as these can produce watery bright yellow stool.

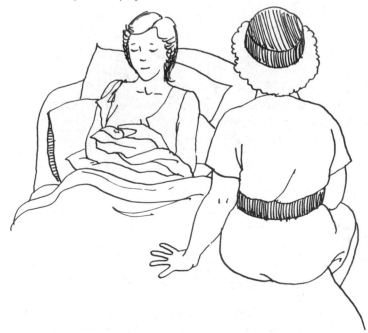

BREASTFEEDING

If the woman is breastfeeding she should be encouraged and boosted in what she is doing, and she should also be told the principles of breastfeeding and how it works.

- That every time the baby sucks she makes milk for him.
- That the more the baby sucks the more milk she will make.
- That the baby knows how long to suck for and how often to suck.
- That if the baby is crying he usually wants to suck.
- That the sucking will become less frequent in time.
- That she will go on producing enough milk for the baby until he is about 9 or 10 months old.
- That there will be times when the baby is growing more quickly than usual and he will cry and cry and want to suck all day, this is because he is building up her milk supply so that it fits his needs.
- That when the baby is about six weeks old her breasts will

go back to their pre-pregnancy size, except that they will have lost some of the fat in them. This means that for a few months her breasts will be soft and floppy, but nonetheless they will be producing pints of milk for her baby. This is important for women to know because the usual reason for women giving up breastfeeding is 'insufficient milk' and this may well be because their breasts feel soft and floppy when in fact they are now lactating very efficiently.

The greatest help to breastfeeding mothers are other women who are also breastfeeding and, as a midwife working in the community, it is important for you to know who runs the local breastfeeding groups or to help a woman start one up. Addresses of the National Childbirth Trust, the La Leche League and the Association of Breastfeeding Mothers are at the back of this book.

Women who are bottle feeding need to be encouraged and shown how to hold the bottle so that the baby is not taking in air with his milk.

Women who are bottle feeding also need to be shown how to mix a bottle to ensure that the way they are doing it is as clean and germ-free as possible. When the midwife arrives in the house she should put the kettle on to boil so that by the time she is ready to mix the bottles the water will be cooling down. Using absolutely boiling water makes the milk lumpy when it is mixed and destroys some vitamins.

The bottles should be kept in a hypochlorite solution for at least one and a half hours prior to being filled (with some tablets this is only 30 minutes), as should the teats. The hypochlorite solution can be kept in a plastic bucket, a plastic ice-cream container or a plastic container specifically produced for sterilising bottles.

Alternatively the bottles and teats can be boiled for five minutes. In both cases the bottles need to have been well cleaned prior to the sterilisation with a bottle brush and detergent.

The mixing of the bottles should take place after the midwife has washed her hands, wiped the work surface to be used and covered it with a clean piece of kitchen roll (if available).

Then show the mother and father how to mix up feeds according to the instructions on the packet.

It is sensible to teach the parents to mix a batch of several feeds at a time because, with all the stresses and strains of new parenthood, it will be very difficult for the mother to get round to mixing feeds when it is appropriate and she will often have a screaming baby and no feeds mixed and maybe no bottles sterilised. Encourage them to change the hypochlorite solution every 24 hours. Made-up bottles should be kept in the fridge until used. They can either be given at room temperature or warmed slightly.

It is essential when showing the mixing of bottles in antenatal classes and in hospital to ensure that the implements used are realistic. The kettle needs to be a real kettle which has actually boiled, the bottles need to have been sterilised in the hypochlorite solution for the requisite time, otherwise women will see that the midwife is using a bottle which was standing unsterilised on the shelf ten minutes ago, that the 'kettle' she is using is actually a jug of warm water and this image will stay with her. This is especially true when the woman is not fluent in the language you are using.

The mother's diet needs to be discussed. Is she eating nutritious foods, does she manage to have time to buy fresh fruits and protein rich foods?

What about rest? How much is she managing to get, or is she trying to be all things to all people – the perfect wife, housewife, hostess as well as mother? The midwife can emphasise to the father that his partner needs to rest, and she can encourage him in his role of taking over domestic chores and childcare.

The essence of good postnatal care is to give the parents confidence in their own abilities. Caplan has shown that the coping response of women to the stresses of childbirth is mainly determined by that woman's innate personality but that the intervention of the care-givers she meets during this time can 'load the dice' either in favour or against the likelihood of her coping well. Jean Ball, in her studies into postnatal depression, shows that the quality of the support the woman receives is extremely important – her main support obviously comes from her family and friends but the support of professionals can make a big difference in enhancing that support.

A few well chosen words from the midwife may be encouraging:

- 'I'm so pleased that you've got some time off work, Stuart. You're cherishing Jean so beautifully – I'm glad you're making sure that she is going to bed for a rest every day.'
- 'It's lovely coming to this house and seeing a new mother being so beautifully looked after.'

The support of professionals can make a difference to the mother herself.

- 'You handle her so well, you've obviously got wonderful mothering instincts – you'd think this was your fourth baby not your first!'
- 'Well done – you do that brilliantly.'
- 'Of course you're tired, it's like being on night duty and when midwives are on night duty they expect to go to sleep all day. *You're* just snatching sleep here and there between Mary's crying. Let's snuggle you down and see if you can get a bit of sleep now, shall we? Your mother-in-law has taken Mary out for a walk. Shall you go and empty your bladder first? – and then I'll talk you through your relaxation and we'll see if you can get off to sleep or at least rest. Having a new baby is really hard work and you're doing it so very well, but the responsibility may get you down at times.'

Sometimes the tiredness is beyond the bounds of physiology and the woman has a full-blown postnatal depression. It is so much easier to spot these if you have been able to form a relationship with the woman before the birth of her baby. Postnatal depression is characterised by a general slow-

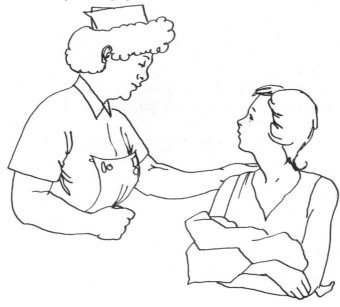

ing down – of movements, reactions, speech, thinking – and a general feeling of not being able to cope, feeling overwhelmed and bleakly despairing. The woman can be helped by organising her family to get her walking every day. Physical exercise can get the whole system moving and adrenaline flowing and can help the woman to improve, as can social contacts and group therapy. Holden (1987) describes the positive effect of eight weekly half-hour counselling sessions from a health visitor on the alleviation of postnatal depression. The description by Van Der Eyken of the work of volunteer visitors on stressed families in the 'Home-Start' scheme also shows the beneficial effect that someone who cares about the woman and provides regular support has on her mental wellbeing. Women experiencing postnatal depression can benefit from psychiatric referral and medication.

Women who have the very frightening experience of puerperal psychosis usually have insomnia, hyperactivity. They can hallucinate, become deranged and paranoid and need urgent psychiatric referral and admission to a specialised mother and baby psychiatric unit. In these cases the husband and family need help and support to cope with the ordeal of seeing a loved relative becoming a total stranger, and they also need to know that the prognosis of this condition is good, that it is self-limiting so that they can go forward with hope.

The health visitor will feature very large in the community midwife's life – it is to her the midwife will turn when she needs to discuss a problem client or when she transfers over a woman who is having problems breastfeeding. It is the health visitor's specialised knowledge of a family having difficulties which can be of enormous help to the community midwife in her work. The health visitor and community midwife can take classes together, run postnatal support groups together, organise breastfeeding support together – it can be an enormously supportive relationship for them both.

Postnatal care can help the family to start parenthood with confidence. It can also be the greatest joy to a midwife, seeing the parents grow in confidence and enjoying their baby. Sharing laughs and experiences with them is a great privilege – intimate moments sitting around the mother's bed can be a time of treasured memories. Sometimes when we sit chatting with these people who have become friends, sipping a cup of coffee and eating cake made by mother-in-law, it is hard to believe that we are being paid to do this – that this lovely experience is called *work*.

References

Ball, Jean, A. (1987). *Reactions to Motherhood: The Role of Postnatal Care*. Cambridge: Cambridge University Press.

Caplan, G. (1964). *Principles of Preventative Psychiatry*. London: Tavistock Publications.

Caplan, G. (1969). *An Approach to Community Mental Health*. London: Tavistock Publications.

Caplan, G., Killilea, M. (1976). *Support Systems and Mutual Help*. Orlando, Florida: Grune & Stratton.

Holden, Jennifer. (1987). She Just Listened. Community Outlook. *Nursing Times*; July.

UKCC. (1986). *Handbook of Midwives' Rules*. London: United Kingdom Central Council for Nursing, Midwifery and Health Visiting, 23 Portland Place, London W1N 3AF. Tel: 01 637 7181.

UKCC. (1986). *Midwife's Code of Practice*. London: United Kingdom Central Council for Nursing, Midwifery and Health Visiting.

Van Der Eyken, Willem. (1982). *Home-Start. A Four-year Evaluation*. Leicester: Home-Start Consultancy.

Chapter Seven

Parentcraft Classes

New parents are embarking upon a totally new phase in their lives, and being aware of this, many choose to come to some form of preparation, both for the coming birth and for the change in their circumstances afterwards. For some people, antenatal classes can be their first brush with 'real' education – education which acknowledges the learner as a unique individual, which acknowledges her influence over her own life and which enables her to change parts of her thinking and pattern of life. 'Real' education is life-changing and leaves the learner a different person from the one who originally stepped through the door of the first session. It is revolutionary for the person experiencing it.

ORGANISING CLASSES

Parentcraft classes and how they are run will vary from area to area. Some people will like to come to a series of classes, others would prefer to drop in on a class from time to time. We write 'people' rather than 'women' because it seems much more sensible to welcome both new parents to the group, if they will come. After all, the life change is great for both of them, though men can be reluctant to come as this scene is not their 'cultural norm'.

How the midwife chooses to organise her classes must depend on her knowledge of the area and the people who live there. If she is starting from scratch it is easiest to discuss with the women she is seeing antenatally what sort of class they would be interested in coming to. At the same time she can be looking around for somewhere to hold the classes. In many health centres there are suitable rooms available for parentcraft classes. Some midwives hold their classes in church halls, and sometimes they can be held in a community centre. All of these venues have the same problem in that they are often impersonal; in such places it is difficult to talk easily about such a personal subject. This will be felt by the participants in the class even more than by the midwife who is leading the group.

Perhaps the best way to start a class is to invite several of the women you are working with antenatally to come to a meeting at a mutually convenient time (when the room you are going to use is free) to discuss pregnancy and labour and then to explore the prospect of life with a baby. You may or may not be in a position to organise a crèche so that other children can be kept entertained while their mothers work in the class. If children are present the group will be subject to many distractions. Sometimes another mother, relative or friend will be willing to babysit.

It is important that the women can sit comfortably, either on the floor (if it is clean) on beanbags or cushions, or on chairs. The person leading the group needs to be sitting at the same level, so if everyone is on the floor the midwife should be too. It is also a good principle that the person leading the group should be dressed in a suitable way to demonstrate different positions in labour and delivery. This may not be very practical in a uniform dress, and uniform may also create a barrier between midwife and woman. Some midwives find themselves too lacking in confidence to take a group without wearing their uniform, but you need to realise that if you wear a uniform it is very likely that you will dominate the group and that is not so helpful for individual learning, even if it makes you feel better.

What have people come for? What can you give them? What is most useful to them and what has been the most permanent benefit? Sometimes the best way to find out what people want from a class is to ask them, but this can't be done if no one has turned up. If there are consistently very few people at your classes or no one, then why aren't people coming to your classes? Could it be that they don't know where and when they are? Or could it be that they are held at a time which is impossible for working women, difficult for women with children already, or out of the question for working men?

People invariably come to parentcraft classes which are offering them what they want, and which they come away from with increased confidence and an awareness that they have learnt from the session.

Having said that, there may be areas where women are housebound. In some cultures it is the women who stay at home and do the cooking and washing while the men do the shopping and go out to work. These women may literally need to be ferried by car to the class. A voluntary group may be willing to take this on, or the hospital care service or even the midwife herself and her colleagues. If the midwife is working with another health professional – such as a physiotherapist or a health visitor – they will need to work closely together and have equal time in the class; but they both need to be there for all the class so that the rhythm of the class is not upset.

WHAT ARE THE CLASSES FOR?

When you are teaching adults *the knowledge is there*. Within the group is all the knowledge that you wish the members of the group to know; all you need to do is unlock it and allow it to flow. You are not trying to teach these people to be mini-midwives, but are there to help them to explore their feelings about the coming change in their life. Between them, three or four adults will have almost all the factual knowledge that you need to impart. They will have learnt it from their mothers, from their friends, from their own experience, from the radio, TV and from magazines and newspapers.

The other, and perhaps the greatest benefit of parentcraft classes, is that of friendship. The people coming to your group are going through the biggest life change most people ever experience. They are going to feel lonely, isolated, sometimes frightened, sometimes overwhelmed. The greatest gift parentcraft classes can give is a friend who is walking the same path, the opportunity to be together with someone rather than doing it all on your own. So the order of priorities for those people coming to a parentcraft class are:

- To make a friend/friends.
- To become aware of their body and how it works.
- To explore feelings about birth and life with a new baby.
- To gain an understanding of the physiology of birth and lactation.
- To get to know what might happen in the hospital.
- To think through strategies for coping with some of the situations which may arise.

MAKING FRIENDS

The way people in a parentcraft class can be helped to make friends is by being given the opportunity to talk – to talk to each other and time to get to know each other. This means that the group leader (you) must learn to be silent and allow the class to talk. This is very difficult for many of us. Midwives are taught by the lecture method and we are used to sitting and listening, and this is what we perceive learning to be: sitting quietly and taking in the knowledge gained from the 'expert' who is lecturing you.

Most of life's skills are not learnt in this way – we learn them from our parents, friends, by looking around ourselves and absorbing what other people are doing, and by exploring our own feelings. The adults who have come to your group are very highly motivated, they have actually come voluntarily to a class, and are expressing their need and willingness to learn and explore. For many people their antenatal classes can be the most exciting educational experience of their lives.

How do we release the knowledge which is there? How do we stay silent and allow it to come out? How can we help the group members to get to know each other?

First, it is important for the group members to know each other's names and for them to have the opportunity to hear each other speak and say something about themselves. Only then will they be able to empathise with another person in the group. Make sure as early on as possible in the group that all the people there have a list of each other's names, addresses and telephone numbers (if they have them). It is

important for you to keep a record of who attends the classes
– an attendance register – for the annual returns of the health
district. They will want to know how many people have
come to the classes which are being provided in their health
authority.

On the subject of making sure the group know each
other's names: this can be achieved by going round the room
and asking each person what their name is, where they are
having their baby, where they live and what they would like
to get out of the classes. It is best to do this in a random order
so that people don't get too het up before they are asked. If
the midwife leading the group gives her full attention to each
person as she asks them the questions the person will then
talk to her and feel less inhibited about the rest of the group.
By the time they leave the class, everyone should know most
people's names, and something about them.

There are also many games designed to help people to get
to know each other, and several excellent books on the subject. Some group leaders have a great repertoire of exercises,
such as getting everyone to say their name and something
about their name, such as, 'I'm Pete, my full name is Pedros
but in English it becomes Pete'; or getting everyone to say
their name and then something about themselves which is
different from anyone else in the room, such as, 'I'm Mary
and this morning I walked the dog for four miles.' If anyone
else in the room walked their dog for four miles that morning
they can challenge Mary and she has to think of something
else unique about herself.

Some group leaders get people to throw a soft ball at each
other and shout out the name of the person who they are
throwing the ball to; others go round the room with the first
person saying 'I'm Margaret' (for example), and the next saying 'I'm Jenny and this is Margaret', and the third giving her
name and the previous two, and so on. Towards the end of
the circle people may need the whole group to help them
remember.

Other leaders ask everyone to say their name and what is
uppermost in their mind at this moment, or what has been

the best thing that has happened to them this week, or the worst thing that has happened to them since the class last met.

These games should be intermingled with other activities designed to enable people to tune into their own bodies and their own feelings. They need to learn to relax, and a good way of splitting up the activities of the class is by having periods of relaxation during the class.

RELAXATION AND SELF-AWARENESS

By learning to relax, people become more aware of their bodies and what is happening inside them. They become aware of their own feelings and they are enabled to tune into their instinctive feelings. Relaxation is a source of great refreshment and tranquillity and having learnt some relaxation techniques the people coming to the class will be able to use their skills

- to surrender and relax during labour, thus enabling the labour to progress as smoothly as possible,
- to tune into their body during labour and to recognise what is happening and how they are feeling,
- to relax after the baby is born when feeding the baby,
- to relax after the baby is born and has been crying and fretful and both parents are exhausted and drained,
- to tune into their instincts after the baby is born and they are worried about something,
- to relax on the day the baby has his first injection or vaccination.

BECOMING AWARE OF YOUR BODY AND YOUR BABY

If you have pillows, or comfortable mats or settees where people can lie supported, that is a great blessing, but you may only have hard chairs and an equally inhospitable floor so there is no way that the group members can loll around or even lie down. This is sad but not insoluble. If people sit with their backs supported they can be helped to relax their whole body and helped to become more aware of it.

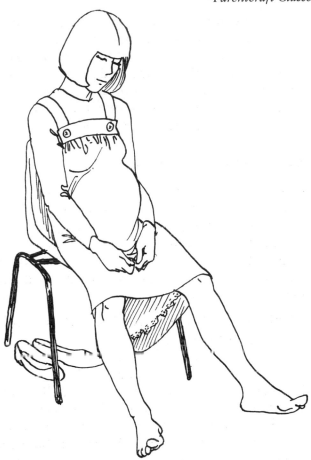

One can start with shutting the eyes.

The group can be made aware of their legs with the chair supporting them underneath their thighs, allowing them to be as rested and relaxed as possible.

The group leader can draw attention to the feet – the toes lying soft and supported in their shoes.

Attention can be drawn up the body, concentrating on the muscles of the pelvic floor, with Kegel exercises being taught. The class members need also to be aware of how stretchy the vagina is with its corrugated sides.

Attention is then turned to the abdominal muscles, tensing

them – almost 'hugging' the baby, and then allowing them to relax so that the baby has more room.

During the relaxation session it is a useful time for the group to think about their baby and how her life is at the moment – snuggled up and comfortable, always cuddled by the uterus, never having known what it's like not to be cuddled, never having known what it's like to be separate and apart, always able to hear the beat of her mother's heart, her breathing, her intestines rumbling, able to hear her mother's and father's voices, not the actual words but the rumbling sound when they speak.

Point out that babies always recognise their mother's voice when they come out. Get the group to think about their baby, always fed, never ever having been hungry, even for a minute, being fed all the time through the umbilical cord, able to drink the amniotic fluid, able to pass urine, suck her thumb, happy when her mother is happy, distressed and upset when she is, afraid when she is – cuddled, well fed, content. Once the parents recognise how their baby is at this time they can more easily realise how different it is for the baby once she is born.

It may help them to appreciate why the baby seems to want to be in their bed with them, why she wants to feed all the time, why she seems lonely and miserable at times. It also makes the class members think of the baby and its personality, which is a useful exercise because many members of parentcraft classes find it difficult to think beyond the birth and the labour. Every opportunity should be taken to think about life with a baby and to lead the expectant parents beyond the birth, because life with a new baby is always such a shock and so very daunting that the new parents can be helped to approach it more realistically by thinking about it beforehand.

The group can be led to think about their spines supported by the chair, and then their arms. Some teachers suggest tensing the muscles of the arm and then comparing the feeling once the arm has been allowed to relax. Others suggest pressing the limbs downwards and then letting go. Whilst doing this the group can be asked how their limbs are feeling and to give words which describe the feelings they are experiencing.

Words which often come are:

Warm
Heavy
Light
Pulsing
Tingling
Comfortable
Supported

Everything a group member says should be affirmed positively. If a group member ever says something completely off beam, she can be affirmed: 'That's an interesting suggestion Desirée, but more often this happens ...' and the more correct interpretation given.

This exercise gives the group the opportunity to really think about a part of their bodies, to explore its feelings and to be aware, sometimes for the first time ever, of what it is like being themselves inside their own bodies. It gives a sense of well being and of being in touch with one's inner self – a sense which many people in our busy world have never had the opportunity to explore. Having asked the group to tell you how it feels for them is a first step to them being able to talk freely within the group, and for them to realise that you expect them to participate fully in these classes.

Everyone has a point where they feel tension more readily than anywhere else and the group, men and women, should be helped to discover their tension points. In labour the women can keep it relaxed and thus keep the whole of their body as relaxed as possible. If men are going to be with their partner during labour they also need to know where her tension point is. They also need to know where their own is, because new babies produce a great deal of tension for both their parents and it's good to teach men how to relax as much as possible.

For many people their place of tension is their shoulders. Get them to lift their shoulders up to their ears, then to drop them slowly as far as possible, then draw their attention to their relaxed shoulders and how they feel. Get the group to listen to their own breathing, and each time they breathe out they are to imagine their shoulders dropping more ... and more ... and more.

Lead the group to focus on their faces and suggest that they keep their eyes shut and screw their faces up into terrible grimaces and then let it go, letting all expression go from the face, letting the lower jaw hang gently, letting the eyelids feel like a great curtain over the eyes, cutting out the light.

The group can be reminded to check on the relaxation of their feet, legs, pelvic floor, abdomens, spines, arms, hands and shoulders and then faces.

The group can then be encouraged to listen to their bodies – to the breath flowing in and out of their lungs, to their heart beating, pumping all the blood round the body. They can sit like this for a minute or two so that everyone can learn to be aware of what it's like being the person inside their body – but state to the group how long you are going to be sitting there in silence otherwise they will think you have gone to sleep and they will be distracted from concentrating on themselves.

This whole exercise needs to be taken through slowly, and it will take up to 20 minutes to go through the whole body. But it is time well spent, for the reasons already given but worth repeating: it will increase the group members' awareness of their bodies, it will help them to be more aware of tension, and it will help them to tune into their own feelings and instincts when the baby arrives. Doing the exercise has also shown them that they are expected to participate in the class. Some kind of relaxation should be done at nearly every class and the group should be encouraged to practise it between the classes too.

EXPLORING FEELINGS ABOUT BIRTH AND LIFE WITH A NEW BABY

The group may be happy about jotting thoughts down on

pieces of paper, but for people who are not at ease with writing and reading it can be too threatening and too reminiscent of school. It is often helpful when exploring feelings and thoughts to split the large group up into little groups of three or four people. In this way people can explore their thoughts in greater privacy and they can also get to know each other more easily.

Some suggestions for discussion topics are:

- Two good things and two bad things about being pregnant.
- Three things my parents did that I shall try to do, and three things which my parents did which I shan't do.
- What I am most afraid of when our labour starts.
- What I'm looking forward to most.
- What my partner/other half is most afraid of about labour.
- What my partner is most hoping for.
- What I am most dreading about life with a new baby and what I am most looking forward to.
- What my partner is most dreading about life with a new baby – what she/he is most looking forward to.

When the small groups have exhausted their discussion (10–20 minutes) then the big group reconvenes and the group leader asks them what they have come up with. The resulting discussion can take anything up to an hour and it will be enormously reassuring for group members to realise that other people feel the same as they do. It will get everyone thinking about their feelings and exploring their thoughts and will be very strengthening. People will also get to know each other more quickly, and friendships built up at this impressionable time often last for the rest of life.

UNDERSTANDING THE PHYSIOLOGY OF BIRTH AND LACTATION

What do people really need to know about?

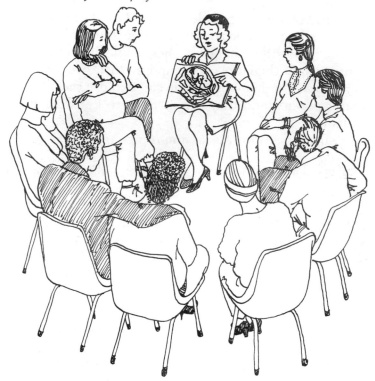

- What is inside their pelvis.
- How the uterus works during labour and dilatation of the cervix.
- What it feels like and ways to help with the pain of labour.

Much of the knowledge which is already within the group can be released by asking questions. For instance, to start a discussion on what is inside the pelvis, you can hold a pelvis close to your own body and ask if anyone knows which organ is immediately behind the symphysis pubis [bladder], sacrum and coccyx [rectum], and get the group to locate the different parts of their pelvis.

How labour starts can be discovered by asking the group how their last labour started – or if they know how labour can start.

Pain relief can be explored firstly by asking them how they

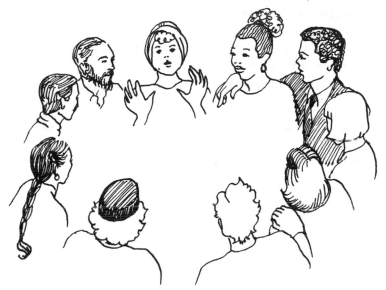

normally cope with pain and discussing that. They may suggest the application of heat or cold, rubbing, walking about, swearing, lying in a warm bath, using a mantra to distract themselves, withdrawing into themselves and concentrating on the centre of the pain, or surrendering totally and letting the pain wash over them.

The most important factor to stress is the length of time it takes for a baby to be born. Most primigravidae experience at least 24–36 hours of labour. Even if we wouldn't classify it as established labour, it feels like labour, and is to all intents and purposes, labour.

After this you could move on by asking the group what they know about the sort of pain relief they may be offered in hospital.

SUGGESTED ORDER OF TOPICS

Most educators would suggest a natural progression for the classes:

1 Pregnancy and its effects (often described best by the men in the group).
2 The end of pregnancy, the loosening effect of progesterone, false labour and how to cope with it.
3 Early labour, through transition and then second and third stage.

As the classes progress so do the subjects. Having got a complete labour into everyone's minds and the baby born, the subjects of analgesia and medically controlled labours can be explored, as can episiotomy, stillborn babies and neonatal death as well as feeding and life with a new baby.

In practice, episiotomy may well come up in Class 1 because someone had a horrible one last time. One might even talk about what it is like to have a stillborn baby because in the first class a woman may tell the group that this is what she experienced last time – or her sister had a stillborn baby last week. When such a topic comes up it needs to be discussed there and then, not left until its planned place in the course. People bring up the things which are troubling them at that moment and if these are not addressed they will not be able to concentrate on other topics.

HELPING THE CLASS ABSORB YOUR TEACHING

In order for people coming to your class to know what they have learnt, tell them at the end of the session. For instance: 'This evening we covered induction and acceleration of labour, the fact that many of you are leaking urine because of the action of progesterone on your pelvic floor muscles, the difficulties of making love when you are so large, the problems that occur when one of you is as randy as hell and the other really doesn't want to know about sex at the moment. The emotional stresses of dealing with relatives crowding in upon you after the birth, and ways to help stitches to heal.'

It also acts as an incentive to tell the group what you will be dealing with next week: 'Next week we shall be talking about caesarean sections and feeding your baby.'

When the group reconvenes it is as well to recap what you did last week – 'Last week we discussed inductions, can anyone remember why they might be done and what they are?' 'And what was acceleration of labour? Why is it done and how is it done?' 'Can anyone remember the effects it is likely to have?'

Having recapped on last week's class, repeat what you are going to teach them this week: 'This week we are going to cover caesarean sections and feeding your baby.'

On the other hand you might find your group is very mobile and likes to discuss whatever comes up. Always finish the class by telling them what topics they covered: it will give them a feeling of satisfaction that they have learnt so much during the session and it will reinforce the learning and help them to retain more.

SOME CONSIDERATIONS IN RUNNING A CLASS

Is your material easy to understand?

Women who are pregnant have a short attention span, 20 minutes of listening is probably the longest they can manage. Their education needs to be broken up into many different sessions:

discussion
listening
relaxing
role playing
drinking tea
more discussion
more relaxing
more listening
more discussion

The use of slides or films

Some teachers use slides depicting a birth. These can be talked through and the group's questions can be explored whilst the slides are being shown. However, many teachers are very wary of films – the image they leave is incredibly strong and if the birth is an idealised one a woman who saw it may feel very disappointed when her experience does not measure up to what she saw in the film. If the birth is particularly gory or old-fashioned questions are stifled during the film because no one likes to interrupt the showing of the film – and then the opportunity is lost after the film has finished because the watchers are too shocked to talk, or too emotional, or the time has passed and the group is on to something else.

For women who do not speak the language that the class is being taken in, slides can be shown very slowly and everything discussed as thoroughly as possible. The same applies in the case of women who are deaf or visually handicapped, who will need the group to explain what they are seeing.

WHAT MIGHT HAPPEN IN THE HOSPITAL

To be fair and honest to women, it is essential to be realistic about what may come their way. What are their chances of having a caesarean section? What are the caesarean section ratios in the hospital they are going to? The epidural rates? The forceps delivery rates? The breastfeeding rates? Women need to be aware of the possibility of caesarean section, induction of labour or augmentation, otherwise, in the event of it happening to them, they feel that somehow they are a freak and that their body has failed to perform as it should. It is worth discussing with women why all these procedures are carried out and ways that the need for them can be minimised.

The most daunting aspect of hospital for many women is the lack of control that they have over anything which may happen to them. Most women are in control of their lives – they decide when they will get up, they decide what they will have for breakfast, they decide whether to go to work or not. Their life is their own to direct as they decide. When they have a baby, especially if it is born in hospital, they will be processed and for the first time in their adult life they will lose control.

For example, could you explore some of the following scenarios in the class?

- The antenatal clinic is on Wednesdays at 2.30 p.m. which is the most inconvenient time of the week for this woman. How can she handle this? Are there any ways of circumventing it?
- The hospital policy is always to give Syntometrine/ Syntocinon/rupture membranes at 4 centimetre, perform routine vaginal examinations every four hours, use continuous electronic fetal monitoring. Are all these beneficial? Does she need to explore what choices she has? If she decides against any of these procedures what can she do?
- The lunch arrives at 12.30 when she has only just started feeding her baby. She'd like lunch in three quarters of an hour instead. Is there anything she can do to enable that to happen? It may be a case of Beryl the domestic goes off duty in half an hour and we've got nowhere to keep your lunch hot. Another mealtime problem may be that she is vegetarian and she has been issued with beef curry. What can she do? Is there any way of being forearmed for these types of frustrations?
- Or perhaps she is asleep and is woken by a midwife because a doctor has come to examine her. Or perhaps she wants to go home this afternoon and there is no doctor to do the required pre-departure examination until tomorrow. What can she do about this?

In an institution the needs of the institution come first, and the needs of both the staff and the women come a very poor second. This may to a certain extent be unavoidable, but if a hotel can cater to the needs of its customers (and staying in a plush hotel costs half the price of keeping someone in a hospital bed) then we suggest that keeping women in hospital should offer the same type of adaptable care that patrons of an hotel receive. If people are being treated for a terrible illness and have faith that they will be cured, or if they have been in pain and are hoping that hospitalisation will help the pain then they will put up with the privations of a hospital routine. On the other hand, women who are having to cope with a huge emotional crisis, who are having to cope with the needs of another human being, a human being who has no idea of mealtimes, sleeptimes, lavatory times or routines, and at the same time are trying to learn a totally new role can find the needs of the institution intolerable. They need to talk to other women who have been through the same experience who can give suggestions for coping with what they are about to cope with.

They need a chance to find out that they can go home whenever they want, and they need to be able to discuss with other mothers the feelings they have had about life with a new baby. To meet this need many midwives are now running postnatal classes as well as antenatal classes. A suggested model might be seven classes before the baby is born and two after the baby is born. The two after the baby is born would take place at a mutually convenient time after all the babies in the group are due to be born.

At the first class everyone could recount their labour, starting with the labour that it's owner felt to be really terrible and ending up with the labour its owner perceived as being the easiest. As this description of labour takes place the teacher or group leader can discover what the group felt unprepared for, what she ought to be adding to her teaching, whether she should be tackling something in a different way.

The second postnatal class can be a discussion of life with a new baby – what everyone needed to know and wasn't prepared for. A common comment is how unprepared they feel for how much time a new baby takes up. It can be helpful in the pre-labour classes to give them a chart (see p. 121) divided up into 24 hours and ask them to fill in how they spent the hours yesterday.

Then give them another chart (see p. 122) and say that they will need to fit around this.

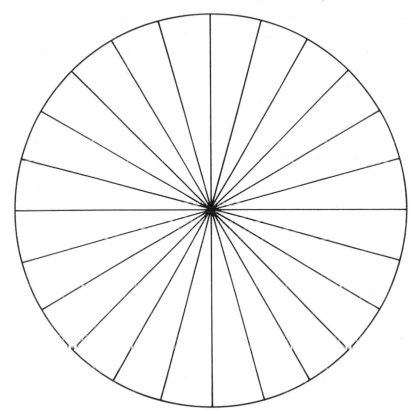

Penelope Leach in her book *The First Six Months* says in her introduction:

'Women-who-become-mothers cannot go on living as they lived before and should not even have to pretend to do so, to outsiders, to their partners, or to themselves. For a while – perhaps for three months, perhaps for two or three times longer – you will find that deep down inside you, nothing matters as much as your baby and nothing which is unimportant to your baby can be very important to you. You will not really be able to tell where "you" end and "the baby" begins because you will feel as if you and she were still part of each other. Even when you are physically away from her, leaving her minute-by-minute care to somebody else, invisible elastic bands will seem to join you together, pulling you back. You are your baby's other half; her

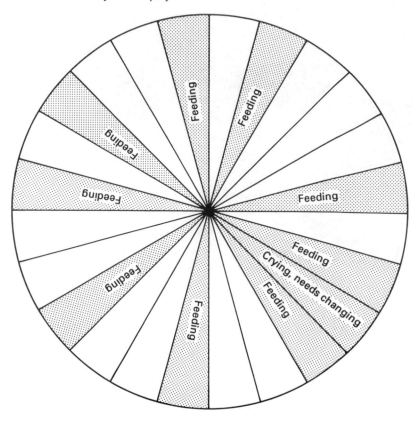

protector, champion and playmate. She is not designed to live without you in these first months. You know it even when nobody else will acknowledge it.'

Some women cannot afford to be this sort of woman, some women do not want to be, but an exploration of how she is likely to feel, and of how, if she lived in many other cultures, she would not be expected to contribute to any other work except for caring for her baby for at least forty days (or six weeks) may help a woman to recognise the pulls of the society she lives in.

Learning that other women are feeling as tied down as she is, as depressed and overwhelmed as she is, as unable to cope as she is, as elated and ecstatic as she is, as besotted by her baby as she is – as aggravated by her husband as she does or as fearful for her husband's safety as she does, is a wonderful relief and helps women to feel strengthened and in control of their world again.

Coming to classes can be an introduction for parents into a new world that can be frightening and demanding, but it can also be a source of strength to cope with the demands being made on them, and a source of friendship and support for starting on the greatest adventure of their lives.

References

Leach, Penelope. (1986). *The First Six Months. Getting Together with Your Baby*. London: Fontana.

Liedloff, Jean. (1975). *The Continuum Concept*. Duckworth and Company Ltd.

Kitzinger, Sheila. (1977). *Education and Counselling for Childbirth*. London: Bailliere Tindall.

Rogers, Jennifer. (1971). *Adults Learning*. Harmondsworth: Penguin Books.

Williams, M., Booth, D. (1974). *Antenatal Education. Guidelines for Teachers*. London: Churchill Livingstone.

Chapter Eight

Equipment

When one looks round any antenatal ward, labour ward, postnatal ward it can seem to the midwife used to working in this environment almost impossible that she can provide herself with adequate equipment that she can carry around with her in her car.

One of the most important pieces of equipment that the midwife will have is in fact her car itself, and it is very worthwhile considering this carefully.

The first decision is whether car ownership or the use of a car provided by the employing authority is going to be the best for you in your practice. There are many things that should be taken into consideration when making this first important decision.

FOR CAR OWNERSHIP

In a practice where one is working in a rural area doing a large mileage and spending a long time in one's car, many of us like to have a car that belongs to us. By and large, mileage allowances will just about cover the costs of car ownership, though some midwives have reported being out of pocket during severe winter conditions with the increased risk of skid damage and the damage that is done by salt and grit.

If one is doing a large amount of 'private' mileage, car ownership is probably better than paying one's employers private mileage rates, which can be quite high.

There is great freedom when one can drive one's own car where and when one wants, without sometimes being required to return it to a base when off-duty.

AGAINST CAR OWNERSHIP

Arguments against car ownership include the difficulties of

security, parking and garaging and the ever-present threat of vandalism in inner-city areas. Many midwives will be unwilling, or unable, to tie up a large sum of money in a car and the necessity to provide one has been a deterrent in many cases in the past to taking a community post.

Recently, employing authorities have introduced schemes whereby community staff are provided with cars under a variety of 'lease car' arrangements. At time of writing these schemes are voluntary for existing employees but could be mandatory for newly appointed personnel. Many of these arrangements are excellent but there can be restrictions placed on the use of the car, and the sum payable to the authority for private use may be considerable, particularly for a person who will do little private mileage, as very often a lump sum is payable for private use.

We suggest that this would be a matter to be explored carefully at interview for any community post and to be taken into serious consideration when making decisions about the acceptability of a job offer. Members of a road-users association will be able to obtain information about comparable car costs from their organisation.

The type of car to have is such an individual choice that there is little point in discussing the merits of different models, though a possible check list of useful attributes could include the following.

- If you will commonly give lifts to pregnant women a four-door car is to be preferred, though if you have small children you may want two doors or very safe childproof locks on the rear doors.
- Do you carry around clipboards, notes, leaflets, etc? If so, nice big shelves under the dashboard, or door pockets, are a boon not just on the driver's side, where they get wet every time you open the door in wet weather, but on the passenger side as well.
- Do you carry equipment for antenatal classes from place to place? A hatchback car with separate split folding-down back seats will be useful to fit the flipchart *and* the projec-

tor *and* the screen *and* the baby bath, and all the other things that find their way into the back of community midwives' cars.

- A sunroof that can be opened easily with one hand is lovely in summer, and a decent heater and demister is a godsend at 3 a.m. in February.
- A trip-meter is useful when calculating one's mileage.
- Two wing mirrors are useful when parking in near impossible spaces or backing into driveways.

A 'midwife visiting' sticker is handy, though inner-city midwives must consider the risk of attracting the attention of those who might be tempted to break in in the hope of finding drugs. A suitable sticker which is recognised by police and traffic wardens can be obtained at moderate cost by sending one's PIN or RCM number to the British Medical Association, Tavistock Square, London WC1 and asking for a sticker.

Incidentally, community midwives should keep the inside of their cars clean and fresh-smelling. The point is that we don't find our own dirt and smells offensive, but many women will be distressed by us entering their homes with dog hairs on our dresses or smelling of our husband's cigarettes. To look professional the vehicle we use needs to look as clean and spick as we should.

EQUIPMENT TO CARRY

The equipment that should be carried to a planned home birth has been described in Chapter 4. Let's now consider what we are likely to find useful and essential as we go on our rounds.

Some of us will prefer to carry a specific antenatal and a postnatal bag, others may use a general bag of useful objects and an attaché case or satchel for the papers, notes and forms. However we carry it, we will need the equipment listed below.

For antenatal care

- A **binaural stethoscope** and a **sphygmomanometer**. If there is any choice over this latter try to get a little aneroid one. They are just as accurate if one takes care to have them serviced regularly, and they are so much smaller and lighter than the mercury metal box type. They are also less prone to damage if dropped or explored by demon toddlers.

- **Reagent sticks** for urine testing. As these sticks are so very sensitive and can show a 'trace' when no actual protein is present, some midwives carry a bottle of salicyl-sulphonic acid and a small test tube to 'cold test' urine for protein. The salicyl-sulphonic acid can be carried in a small, dark-coloured poison bottle with a dropper stopper, which with a small test tube can fit nicely into a plastic soap container. Some cotton wool stops it rattling around and would absorb the small amount of acid spilled if the stopper became loose. The bottle, of course, is clearly labelled.

  The method is to place about 2–3 cm of urine in the test tube, and add a few drops of salicyl-sulphonic acid. If albumin is present the urine will become cloudy.

- A **Pinard's stethoscope**. The wooden ones are kinder to the ears and the maternal abdomen in cold weather and they don't seem to conduct the other noises – traffic, television, animals – that the metal ones do. (They are obtainable from Association of Radical Midwives, 62 Greetby Hill, Ormskirk, Lancs.)

  If you ever find yourself needing to listen to a fetal heart without a stethoscope, a cardboard loo-roll holder makes an excellent substitute. The midwife's ear can always be applied direct to the abdomen, of course, but not every woman likes this.

- A **portable fetal heart monitor** is nice to have if you can persuade your authority to supply one. Many midwives employed by penniless authorities and lacking such an item, have persuaded local charitable organisations such as Round Table, Soroptomists, or morris dancers to raise money to buy them one. Whether one should be dependent on charity for such things is an ideological question beyond the scope of this book.

- The appropriate **forms**, and **containers, syringes, needles** and a **tourniquet** to take blood for antenatal tests.
- **Maternity benefit information** and the appropriate **application forms.**
- **Containers for varous specimens** e.g. urine for microbiology.
- **Swab sticks** and **transport media** for the various specimens obtained for bacteriological examination.
- A **'sharps' disposal container.**
- A **tape measure**, useful for measuring abdominal girth in cases of suspected polyhydramnios, or postnatally to compare calf girth in cases of suspected deep vein thrombosis.
- A **good torch**, used for everything from finding house numbers at night to inserting or removing perineal sutures!
- **Sterile disposable gloves**, a sterile **lubricant**, and sachets of suitable **lotion for vulval swabbing** should also be carried for the antenatal visit made to assess if a woman is in, or how she is progressing in, labour.

For postnatal care

- A **thermometer.** Some of us will have a supply of thermometers which we will leave in each house, collecting them on our last visit. Traditionally they were stood in an empty fish paste pot in some dilute disinfectant. This is a quite dangerous thing to do and very poor teaching for the parents to leave a container of disinfectant around where it could be imbibed by children, either of the household or visiting. After use, the thermometer can be cleaned by cold running water and dried and left in the Notes envelope. It also provides the opportunity for teaching parents about thermometer use and care.
- A pair of **'nursing'** scissors for cutting off namebands, opening sachets and a hundred and one other uses.
- **Equipment to remove perineal sutures.** There are some

very nice presterilised suture removal packs available, containing a suture removal scalpel, some sterile gauze swabs, a pair of plastic dissecting forceps and a plastic disposal bag.

One could alternatively carry a pair of sharp scissors and a pair of dissecting forceps. If this equipment is chosen it is important that satisfactory arrangements are available for sterilising, either an arrangement with one's local CSSD department or the use of an autoclave at a convenient health centre. The use of so-called sterilising fluids cannot be recommended.

- A **Cuscoe's speculum** for taking high vaginal swabs. Again there are presterilised disposable ones available. If non-disposable ones are used the comments on sterilisation above apply.

- **Glycerine suppositories** are useful for the relief of the constipated woman with a painful perineum. A small pack can be carried which can be bought cheaply at any chemist.

- **Something for the relief of perineal pain.** Every community midwife will have her own pet remedies and suggestions for the relief of perineal pain. Equipping oneself with a sympathetic ear and a realisation of just how miserable this can be for the woman is essential.

An old-fashioned remedy is Lotio Rubra (Red Lotion): zinc sulphate 1% in water with amaranth 1 ml in 100 ml. A sterile swab soaked in this and applied to painful perineal wounds is reported by many women to be soothing. It is also helpful in cleaning the broken down episiotomy wound. The hospital pharmacy can be asked to make it up, or it can be prescribed by general practitioners on S.P. 10.

There are many other preparations which midwives may suggest. Among them Arnica, either the lotion or the ointment. This is further discussed in Chapter 6.

- The midwife could also carry in her bag **a preparation for the treatment of prolapsed piles**, which frequently seem to need urgent treatment at weekends or bank holidays. A word of warning here. Experienced midwives have found that where there are catgut perineal sutures several of the proprietary haemorrhoidal preparations appear to accelerate the breakdown of catgut.

- A **small breast pump** can be useful in some cases, used gently to relieve milk engorgement or to gently draw out retracted nipples before assisting with 'fixing' on the breast. It is also useful to carry one to teach the correct use to the mother who may be returning to work, but who wishes to continue feeding.
- It is useful to carry a **small bottle of antiseptic hand-rub** for use in the home where hand washing using the facilities available is unlikely to improve the cleanliness of one's hands.
- In the right-hand top corner of our bags there is a red plastic soap box containing a **2 ml syringe**, an **intramuscular needle**, an **injection swab**, an **ampoule of 0.5 mgm ergometrine** and an **ampoule of Syntometrine 1 ml**. The ampoules are separately taped down to the bottom of the box with narrow 'sellotape'. They are instantly accessible should they be required urgently for the emergency treatment of postpartum haemorrhage. We suggest that each community midwife should carry such an emergency package always in the exact same place in her equipment. It is important to remember to check the expiry dates of these drugs.

For baby postnatal care

- Some **sachets of sterile normal saline** for swabbing 'sticky' eyes. It is useful to carry this because not all mothers will be able to follow instructions for making up the following solution at home. Take a one pint bottle, clean it very thoroughly. Sterilise it with hypochlorite solution (the chemical used in all feeding bottle sterilizing tablets and liquids) and fill it with previously boiled water. To this add one teaspoonful of household salt. This gives 0.9% solution adequately accurate for this purpose. If a clean egg-cup or small glass is upturned over the bottle it can be used

as a galley pot every time the eyes are swabbed. The solution should be renewed daily.
- **Swabs transport media** for bacteriological testing.
- **Equipment for testing serum bilirubin.**
- **Mucus extractors.** Rarely one has a mucosy baby and it is sometimes wise to teach the parents how to 'suck out' the baby and leave a mucus catheter in the house for the parents to use. The midwife's skills will be needed in assessing the abilities of parents to cope with this responsibility and to learn the technique.
- **Guthrie cards and lancets** for heel pricking. It is a good idea to do this test with the baby in the mother's arms, for the imagination can often be much worse than the reality and many mothers whose babies are taken away to have this and other tests done in hospital imagine all sorts of things. The mother who is reluctant to be involved can be helped to a realisation of her importance to her baby, and of how much comfort her loving arms will bring to her child throughout all the traumas of childhood, perhaps starting with the Guthrie test and going on to the immunisations, the falls, knocks and bumps of toddlerhood, and the problems of childhood.
- **Baby weighing scales,** Which often tell us what we know already about a baby's condition but which can be helpful either to confirm that a baby is indeed failing to thrive or to confirm to a mother that her baby is thriving. Very accurate spring balance ones can be bought in angling shops. Anglers need to have scales that are accurate to the last ounce to ensure that their fishy competitions (and stories) have credibility!

Other equipment

Other equipment that midwives might like to carry could include:

- A box containing two **intravenous-giving sets** and **500 ml bags of intravenous fluid,** such as dextrose 5% and a bag of Hartmann's solution. These are carried so that they are available in an emergency for a medical practitioner to use or, in the absence of a medical practitioner, for the midwife to use. One of us recollects using IV equipment in an emergency situation: an antepartum haemorrhage in a hospital-booked case. This occurred on a bank holiday Saturday in a popular holiday resort. The flying squad had great difficulty getting through the traffic. A local GP and the midwife were able to use the equipment carried by the midwife, so that when the ambulance did eventually get there, there was a vein open, and an IV *in situ*. Even though the APH was quite severe, resuscitation was more speedy and effective than if collapsed veins had had to be overcome.

- A small stock of **inco pads** and **sanitary pads** have a multitude of uses. The most unusual use for inco pads that either of us remember is putting them under the wheels of the midwife's car stuck in a snowdrift!

- We require **communication equipment**. Fortunate midwives will have two way radio telephones. Most of us will have some form of 'bleep'. We must remember that in the past midwives often did not even have telephones and had to leave messages all over the place concerning their whereabouts. Often homes were not on the telephone, and older midwives will remember making arrangements involving nappies hung in windows and messages relayed through postmen and milkmen. In one area one of us remembers a box in the local police station where messages could be left for the midwife. We have more efficient and reliable means of communication now but it is just as important as it ever was that we ensure that the methods by which we can be reached are reliable and carefully explained and understood.

The supervisor of midwives has the right and the duty to inspect our equipment. Community midwives have a duty to ensure that their equipment is adequate, and regularly reviewed, renewed, and serviced. The supervisor should be informed and her advice and guidance sought if the midwife encounters any difficulty in maintaining supplies or having maintenance of equipment carried out.

Supervisors are commonly managers of midwifery services. We can often assist them when they are making bids for funding for equipment, for both community and institutional services, if we state clearly to them, preferably in writing, what we need to enable us to deliver a high standard of care. So often one hears that expensive equipment can be obtained for the hospital but the community service struggles with what it has got. Perhaps this could be our own fault. We have been so intent in providing the service, getting the visits done, 'covering' the clinics, that we have neglected to make our need for supplies and improved equipment quite clear to those responsible.

Chapter Nine

The Community Midwife and the Law

The law relating to midwives is enshrined in the Nurses, Midwives and Health Visitors Act 1979. This Act repeals the Midwives Acts of 1902, 1918, 1926, 1936 and 1951 and enabled the setting up of the United Kingdom Central Council for Nursing, Midwifery and Health Visiting (UKCC). The UKCC provides for the education, training, regulation and discipline of nurses, midwives and health visitors. The Act at the same time sets up national boards for each country within the UK.

The 1979 Act describes the functions of the Council and allows for the giving of professional advice to nurses, midwives and health visitors and this can be a very useful aspect of the Council's functions. At the Council there is a professional officer for each specialty. If you are ever having problems regarding your professional practice and you are needing encouragement, or advice, it is well worth contacting the professional officer (midwifery) at the UKCC.

As well as setting up the Council and describing its functions the Act prescribes the registration of all nurses, midwives and health visitors, lays down the rules regarding the training of midwives – the length of training, the age of entry and examinations etc., and also describes removal from or restoration to the register.

The UKCC is directed by law to make rules regulating the practice of midwives – thus the Midwives' Rules are emanations from the Act and are the law of the land. The Rules are particularly concerned with the suspension of midwives from practice, notification of intention to practise and attendance at refresher courses.

It is essential for every midwife in practice to have a copy of the Midwives' Rules. They are available from the United Kingdom Central Council, 23 Portland Place, London W1N 3AF (Tel: 01 637 7181) at a nominal cost (£1 in 1987).

The aspect of the Rules which concern the midwife practising in the community, either as an employee of the National Health Service or as a self-employed independent practitioner, are those relating to practice.

The Rules define the requirements of midwives to notify their 'Intention to Practise' before they practise or within 48 hours of having practised, and to fill in a notification of intention to practise in March of each year. The Rules also specify that a midwife should attend a refresher course every five years.

The Rules then specify those reasons for which a midwife may be suspended from practice and the procedure relating to preventing the spread of infection. Suspending a midwife from practice is an extremely serious step as it withdraws from the midwife concerned her professional status. It can only be done (except in the need for preventing the spread of infection) after the Local Supervising Authority (the Regional Health Authority in England) has either reported the midwife to the investigating committee of the appropriate national board, or after the midwife has been referred to the Professional Conduct Committee of the UKCC, or after the midwife has been referred to the Health Committee of the Council.

The reason that this step is so serious is that once the midwife has been referred to an investigating committee and then to the professional conduct committee, the only power the professional conduct committee has is that of removing the name of the midwife from the register. Obviously the whole system should never be put into motion unless what the midwife has done is so serious that she should be struck off the register. Thankfully, the other power the professional conduct committee has is to take no action.

It is only the local supervising authority which can suspend a midwife from practice and not a supervisor of midwives. So, if a supervisor of midwives tells you that she is suspending you from practice, she is acting incorrectly and you should refer her to the Midwives' Rules. If she is your employer she can suspend you from duty – but this is in her role as employer not as supervisor.

THE INVESTIGATING COMMITTEE

The investigating committee of each national board looks at each case which is referred to it – and once a midwife has been referred to the investigating committee the case cannot be stopped because the referrer has changed her mind. Once the system has been instituted it has to be seen through.

Immediately the board receives a case against a midwife to go before the investigating committee, an officer of the board writes to the midwife concerned and tells her what the allegations against her are and asks her to send a statement to answer these charges. The investigating committee looks at allegations of professional misconduct from colleagues, managers, mothers, their relatives, or any private citizen. They then study the documentation they have received, they read what the professional has written in mitigation and then they take any one of four steps:

- No action.
- Referring the practitioner to the code of practice and saying that they consider that professional misconduct could have occurred but is not proven.
- Referral to the professional conduct committee.
- Referral to the health committee.

PROFESSIONAL CONDUCT COMMITTEE

The professional conduct committee, which is made up of five members of the UKCC and an experienced lawyer to advise on the law and to ensure the proper conduct of the hearing, has, first of all, to ascertain that what the professional has been accused of did actually happen. They hear evidence from both sides and they can subpoena witnesses if necessary.

If they decide that the episode did not happen the case stops and the file is destroyed.

If they decide that it did happen, they then decide whether it was misconduct in a professional sense.

If it wasn't misconduct the case stops, and the file is destroyed. If it was misconduct, they ask the accused for evidence in mitigation, so that the person accused can show any reasons why she acted in the way she did.

The committee then retires to decide on their judgement and the actions available for them to take are:

- To take no action.
- To take no action but refer the practitioner to the *Code of Professional Conduct.*
- To postpone judgement until a future date.
- To remove from the register.

The details of the case are kept on file for many years.

The Rules set out the responsibility and sphere of practice of the midwife:

'A practising midwife is responsible for providing midwifery care to a mother and baby during the antenatal, intranatal and postnatal periods. In any case where there is an emergency or where she detects in the health of a mother and baby a deviation from the norm a practising midwife shall call to her assistance a registered medical practitioner, and shall forthwith report the matter to the local supervising authority in a form in accordance with the requirements of the local supervising authority.'

There can be instances where, as a midwife working in hospital, you would refer to a doctor because he is just outside the door and very accessible, and where at home you have a problem doing this.

For instance, you may be attending a home birth where you have a very unsympathetic GP who wants nothing to do with the delivery. You detect meconium-stained liquor but, because the meconium staining is only slight and you are nearly in second stage, and the fetal heart is all right, you feel that you can deal with it at home. In another instance, the woman has a postpartum haemorrhage and you deal with it at home and don't see any necessity to take her into hospital. You are obliged by the Rules to 'call to your assistance a registered medical practitioner' in both cases. It is however obvious that you cannot and do not want to call an unwilling and probably not very useful GP, especially when it is a situation which you have already dealt with. It seems ridiculous to call the local hospital and speak to the registrar on call to say, 'I'm just waking you up at 3 o'clock in the morning to say that I am a midwife looking after a woman called Mary Rakes (who you don't know) at home. She delivered an 8 lb 10 oz baby boy an hour ago and had a postpartum haemorrhage following his birth. She lost 1,000 ml of blood, I gave her Syntometrine, delivered the placenta, catheterised her to empty her bladder, her blood pressure is 100/60, her pulse is 84, she is no longer bleeding and, although she is feeling shaky she seems in a stable condition. I am keeping an eye on her for the next two to three hours but I don't think I shall transfer her to hospital. I'm just letting you know because in my Rules it says I must and now that I've woken you, you can lie awake and worry about it.' The best alternative is to ring the supervisor of midwives to let her know what is happening, and to gain her advice and supportive counsel.

The difficulty of course is when the supervisor of midwives is not clinically up-to-date and she may just panic at the situation you are describing and order you to transfer the woman to hospital, which may not be in the best interests of the woman or her baby. Often midwives are in Catch 22 situations – clinical midwives in our society at the moment are invariably managed, led, judged by and sentenced by midwives who are no longer clinicians.

'A practising midwife must not, except in an emergency, undertake any treatment which she has not been trained to give either before or after registration as a midwife and which is outside her sphere of practice.'

The important words here are 'except in an emergency' – so if you have a woman who is bleeding and you put up an intravenous infusion of Haemaccel whilst waiting for the ambulance or flying squad to arrive, you are acting in an emergency. If you put up an intravenous infusion when there is no emergency you are acting outside your sphere of practice.

As far as recording of information goes:

'A practising midwife shall keep as contemporaneously as is reasonable detailed records of observations, care given and medicine or other forms of pain relief administered by her to mothers and babies.'

In other words the midwife keeps a diary of what is happening and what she is giving to or doing to the woman and baby, which she writes as she goes along. This obviously means that sometimes the notes are in the thick of the action and they get slightly blood-spattered or wet with amniotic fluid.

There are two ways of looking at the writing of notes. Firstly, obviously the better way is to write down each and everything which happens, but it needs to be acknowledged that this can intrude in your relationship with the woman and her partner. If this road is followed the midwife and the woman have a permanent record of what happened at the birth of each baby. On the other hand if a supervisor of midwives or doctor is feeling litigious against the midwife, it is always possible to pore through notes and find areas which can be criticised with the benefit of hindsight, in the sphere of clinical practice.

The other way of writing notes, which some practitioners follow because of bitter experiences, is effectively to write nothing, either literally or more infuriatingly:

11/2/89 10.15 a.m. All observations normal.
11/2/89 10.30 a.m. All observations normal.
11/2/89 11.00 a.m. Labour progressing well.

Very different from:

11/2/89 10.15 a.m. Mary is on all fours on a soft mat, she is groaning with contractions which are coming every 3 minutes and are strong, but she is actually remaining very relaxed and content through them. Fetal heart heard with Sonicaid and is regular at 136 beats per minute. John is lying underneath Mary and wiping her face with a cool flannel and saying comforting words to her.

11/2/89 10.30 a.m. Mary is staggering to the bathroom helped by John because I have suggested that being in the bath might help at this stage. She is stopping at the lavatory on the way and has passed urine (not measured or tested because it is too awkward).

11/2/89 11 a.m. Mary has spent the last half hour in the bath with much benefit. The fetal heart has been checked twice during this period and both times was regular and between 136 and 140 bpm.

The notes are legal documents and must be preserved by the midwife and given to the local supervising authority just before she ceases to practise. In her will she must leave instructions to her executors about her notes, or instructions to her relatives in case of her having an accident or being killed.

INSPECTION OF PREMISES AND EQUIPMENT

The midwife must allow the supervisor of midwives access to her methods of practice, her records, her equipment and such part of her residence as may be used for professional purposes. This means that the supervisor of midwives can ask to see where you keep your equipment and you must show her the cupboard where you keep it, but it doesn't mean that she must be shown round the house or ask to inspect the kitchen or the horror of the teenagers' bedrooms.

If you have women to stay when they have their babies you are using your home as a nursing home and specific regulations apply, details of which can be obtained from reading the Nursing Homes Registration Act available from HMSO.

The Midwives' Rules lay upon you an obligation to fill in a Notification of Intention to Practise form once a year in every health authority you intend to practise as a midwife in. To obtain this you write to the local supervisor of midwives c/o the head of maternity services at the local maternity hospital. If you have problems finding out who your local supervisor of midwives is, telephone the regional health authority and ask to speak to whoever acts as the local supervising authority. In rural districts you will probably only have an Intention to Practise form to fill in for one or two districts, but in the metropolitan areas each midwife may have more Intentions to Practise to take out and consequently more supervisors of midwives. It is important to keep these up to date – they need to be renewed every March.

The other obligation that the Midwives' Rules lay upon you is to attend a refresher course every five years. For community midwives the cost is borne by your health authority but if you are working part-time you may have to negotiate with your employers to try and persuade them to finance you. The refresher courses get overbooked extremely quickly and you may want to go to a specific course, such as the Research Appreciation Refresher Course put on by the Royal College of Midwives or a course put on by a college that you know is good. In order to have any choice in where you go for your course, you need to take steps during the preceding year to find out what choices you have and to obtain a list of the courses from the professional officer at the English National Board (address on p. 240). She keeps a list of all the refresher courses because they have to be approved by the Board. Many of the refresher courses are run by the Royal College of Midwives (address on p. 241), who publish a list of the ones they are running for the next year by September of the previous year. In order to ensure a place on the course you wish to go on you should book up a place the preceding September, and claim the money back from your health authority later. This presupposes that you have about £250 spare, which may not be the case. For self-employed midwives the cost of refresher courses is tax deductible. There are moves to enable midwives to accumulate approved study days over a period of five years.

Obviously as a person with a professional qualification needing to retain credibility, it is important to keep professionally up-to-date. The easiest way to achieve this is to subscribe to as many magazines and journals as possible and especially to MIDIRS, which enables you to read a selection of different papers from different journals. It is a good idea systematically to visit a medical library at regular intervals and read through the articles which interest you, perhaps the third Thursday of each month or another specific day. Most supervisors of midwives will be able to arrange access for you to the nearest medical library. With recent facts and figures under your belt you will feel more confident, and you will provide women with a richer service, based on knowledge and research findings as well as on intuition and good will, which, while they are important are only a part of being a midwife. Throughout the country excellent study days and conferences are held. It is worth looking out for them and requesting study leave, and perhaps finance, in order to attend them.

A MIDWIFE'S CODE OF PRACTICE

This is available free of charge fom the UKCC (address p. 151). It elaborates on the Midwives' Rules and contains guides to good practice for midwives. It is not the law of the land but is very much taken into consideration by the UKCC when they are looking at complaints about a midwife's practice.

The Code of Practice starts off by saying:

> 'Each midwife as a practitioner of midwifery is accountable for her own practice in whatever environment she practises. The standard of practice in the delivery of midwifery care shall be that which is acceptable in the context of current knowledge and clinical developments.'

(Thus the need to keep up-to-date and to read as much as you can.)

The Code of Practice then goes on to give the definition of a midwife from the World Health Organisation, the International Confederation of Midwives and the International Federation of Gynaecologists and Obstetricians:

'A midwife is a person who, having been regularly admitted to a midwifery educational programme, duly recognised in the country in which it is located, has successfully completed the prescribed course of studies in midwifery and has acquired the requisite qualifications to be registered and/or legally licensed to practise midwifery.

She must be able to give the necessary supervision, care and advice to women during pregnancy, labour and the postpartum period, to conduct deliveries on her own responsibility and to care for the newborn and the infant. This care includes preventative measures, the detection of abnormal conditions in mother and child, the procurement of medical assistance and the execution of emergency measures in the absence of medical help. She has an important task in health counselling and education, not only for the patients, but also within the family and the community. The work should involve antenatal education and preparation for parenthood and extends to certain areas of gynaecology, family planning and child care. She may practise in hospitals, clinics, health units, domiciliary conditions or in any other service.'

The Code then continues with a list of competencies required of a midwife. It then lists how a midwife should practise in her administration of drugs, destruction of controlled drugs and what to advise a woman who has obtained an ampoule of a controlled drug (such as pethidine) for her home confinement and has not used it and wishes to dispose of it. The Code also details the legislation for supplying prescription only drugs to midwives – this is useful to have listed for when a midwife needs to go to a dispensing chemist to obtain such drugs as Syntometrine, ergometrine, intravenous Haemaccel or chloral hydrate tablets.

The Code expands on notifying an Intention to Practise and then goes on to home confinements. Here it states that when a registered medical practitioner is not available to attend (if required), the midwife must inform the supervisor of midwives. Sometimes the supervisor will find a registered medical practitioner who is willing to be called if required, but often she just arranges with the midwife that in case of any illness or abnormality of the mother, fetus or baby, the midwife will transfer the patient to the local maternity unit.

If a woman decides to have a home birth and the midwife advises that it is, in her opinion, medically inadvisable to have a home birth, obviously the woman can either act on or ignore that advice. If she ignores the advice the midwife must continue to give care to the woman but she must inform her supervisor of midwives. In this case, the supervisor would telephone occasionally to give the midwife moral support and would alert the flying squad just in case. She might also send another midwife (if the woman agreed) to give the original midwife moral support.

Such an instance occurred when Caroline booked Flo for a home delivery. It was Flo's second baby and her pregnancy progressed normally and happily, but at 34 weeks the baby was in a breech position, and remained breech at 36 weeks. Caroline advised Flo that delivering a baby in a breech position was not considered a normal delivery and that there were greater risks for the baby in such a birth – which she detailed – and consequently she advised Flo to have the baby in hospital. Flo said 'No thank you', so Caroline arranged with the local supervisor of midwives that if Flo went into the local hospital the obstetric team would deliver her baby and she could come out immediately after the birth. Flo again said 'No thank you'. Caroline arranged with another supervisor of midwives and one of the obstetricians in her unit that Caroline could take Flo into hospital, deliver Flo herself with obstetric and paediatric back-up and bring Flo and her baby home again immediately after delivery. Flo again said 'No thank you', and said quite categorically that she was having her baby at home. Caroline informed the local supervisor of midwives and carried on looking after Flo in accordance with Rule 4(b). A GP was willing to come to the delivery to aid with resuscitation if necessary (she ended up as camera woman) and another midwife came to support Caroline and to give expertise. The birth turned out to be a wonderful experience for the parents and for all the professionals involved and the baby looked quite pleased with herself too when she arrived! Perhaps the moral of the story is: teamwork, liaison and DON'T PANIC!

If a midwife wants to call a doctor and the woman refuses to allow this, the midwife must again continue to give care and inform her supervisor of midwives. This is not as clear cut as it sounds. Sometimes when the midwife goes to ring the GP who has asked to be there for second stage of labour, the woman will say 'Oh no, don't ring him, it's so cosy being here just the three of us.' The midwife cannot then ring the GP. In theory she should at that time telephone the supervisor, but she is usually too occupied with the imminent delivery to be able to telephone the hospital, which involves waiting five minutes for the switchboard to answer and than another five for the supervisor to be located. So it is practical for her to do it afterwards.

The Code of Practice states that whenever a midwife employs a substitute to attend a woman in childbirth it must be either a registered medical practitioner or a registered midwife. It details that the midwife must inform the supervisor of midwives in the case of a maternal death, neonatal death or stillbirth occurring.

The equipment of a midwife practising in the community or in independent practice should be specified by the local supervising authority or by the supervisor of midwives on behalf of the local supervising authority. It is worth keeping an eye on what is specified because many health authorities supply the very minimum to their midwives because of the expense. Most independent midwives appear to be better equipped than their NHS counterparts.

The Code lists the definition of live and stillborn babies:

'A baby born at any stage of pregnancy who breathes or shows other signs of life after complete expulsion from its mother is **born alive**. If such a baby dies after birth, the birth and death will both require to be registered.'

'A baby who has issued forth from its mother after the 28th week of pregnancy and has not at any time after being completely expelled from its mother breathed or shown any sign of life is a **stillborn baby.**'

'The birth before the 28th week of pregnancy of a baby who did not breathe or show signs of life after complete expulsion from its mother is **neither a live birth nor a stillbirth** and need not be registered.'

The Code also lists and summarises other relevant legislation which affects midwives, including exemption from jury service.

REGISTERS

Every midwife is required to have in her possession two registers, both available from Hymns Ancient and Modern (address p. 151). *Registers of Cases I* is to record each day of the year and to list what visits a midwife made on each day, either antenatal or postnatal visits, or visits which were unsuccessful because the woman was out. It is a good idea to keep this register in your car and fill it in as you progress through your visits. The squares in it are rather difficult to distinguish and it can be very helpful to highlight the Saturdays and Sundays so that you can easily ascertain which day you are on, otherwise the squares dance around in front of your eyes (this may be the subjective feelings of two middle-aged women, those with younger eyes may not have this problem).

Register of Cases II is a record of personal deliveries. It can be very pleasant to keep a record of every baby delivered, and the Register can be adapted to keep more information than at first there seems place for.

The register has sections under which it lists:

Number
Patient's name and the address where delivery takes place. It is as well also to list here the woman's home address, her partner's name and her telephone number.

Age

Date of booking. Many midwives add length of pregnancy in this space.

Expected date of delivery

Number of previous labours and miscarriages. Pregnancies are usually listed as T = 1 (One Termination) M = 0 (no Miscarriages) L2 (Two Labours) or Gravida 4 Para 3.

Date and hour of midwife's arrival, to which can be added the length of labour. There is room to detail the length of each stage with the total:

9:15 (First stage was 9 hours and fifteen minutes)
1:06 (Second stage was 1 hour and 6 minutes)
0:09 (Third stage was 9 minutes)
10:30 (Total length of labour was 10 hours 30 minutes)

Date and hour of infant's birth

Sex of infant, alive or dead. Here it is useful to include the baby's first name.

Birth weight

Then there is a very small unmarked column. This can be used for blood group, if required, or type of onset of labour.

Persons present other than the midwife

Date of transfer to the health visitor. To this can be added perineal trauma.

Date of last visit – to which can be added Apgar score and condition of baby at birth.

Drugs given: date and time of administration

Other information can include: type of onset; a brief summary of the labour; type of delivery and position of baby; blood loss; details of alternative positions or how the baby was delivered; how the membranes ruptured and how the third stage was conducted.

At the end of each year it is an idea to gather statistics of how your deliveries went, how much analgesia you used, how many women had intact perineums or 1st or 2nd degree tears.

A midwife's work diary is as useful as her registers in ascertaining her practice and is looked upon as a legal document. It also needs to be kept carefully with the notes and registers that the midwife keeps.

CONFIDENTIALITY

It seems easy to protect confidentiality, but attention must be given to it.

'How's Joan, what did she have?'
'A little girl.'
'How did everything go?'
'Well, she had a long labour and after 16 hours she was finding the pain too much so I transferred her to hospital, she had an epidural and then a normal delivery. I needed to give her an episiotomy and her stitches are a bit sore especially as she's got piles. She's very weepy because she wanted to have the baby at home and I think she's exhausted as well because the baby's crying a lot ...'

So now the old lady who lives next door to Joan knows that Joan has piles, is weepy, found the pain of labour very great, had an epidural and had stitches. Joan may be a very private person and her private details have no business being discussed by the midwife. Try again:

'How's Joan, what did she have?'
'She had a baby girl.'
'How did everything go?'
'Well of course I can't discuss it, but she did very well.'

Confidentiality needs to be part of your life. It is easy to come home after an exciting delivery and detail the whole of it to your best friend. This is probably all right if she is in the same profession, but care needs to be taken otherwise you may be at a dinner party and you may hear your husband at the other end of the table chiming out with, 'Oh yes, Sylvia had a very interesting case the other day when the woman wanted to give birth squatting, but her husband had an argument with her because he found it strained his hands if he supported her in that position...' Or even worse: 'Mum, I told Mrs Simpkins (teacher) that you had looked after a woman who didn't like midwives and that she had shouted at you that she would set the dogs on you. I also told Mrs Simpkins that your boss is a pig and Mrs Simpkins was very sorry for you.'

A more shady area is when you take antenatal classes. Joyce rings up and tells you a blow by blow account of her labour, or you deliver Joyce and the rest of the class want to know how everything went. It is essential to ask Joyce how much you should tell her class mates, or even better if she or her partner can come to the next class and give their own summary.

Every midwife has anecdotes; these are extremely pleasant to tell and hear and they are useful for others to learn from, but it is essential that the woman's identity is disguised or you will be in the embarrassing position of someone saying: 'Oh I know her, we go to yoga together, I'll tell her I met her midwife when I go tomorrow.'

Another ethical problem arises when you are in a woman's home and when you dry your hands you are given a towel with 'St Margaret's Hospital' firmly written on it. The baby is dressed in 'hospital property' and the sheets on the baby's crib are similarly marked. A useful way to deal with this can be to say: 'I'll take these back to the hospital, shall I? If you bundle them up I'll collect them all tomorrow.' It can be helpful to keep a collection of 'nearly new' baby clothes which you can give to women who are short of clothes for their baby, or short of the money to buy clothes with. Once people know that you would like some baby clothes you will be surprised how many you will receive.

The midwife will find herself confronted by dilemmas for which there are no easy answers. For instance, the midwife knows that this woman's husband has had homosexual lovers, the wife doesn't appear to know, the midwife wonders if her information could be faulty. Can she ask the woman if she might be at risk of AIDS? Can she ask her if she would like to be tested for AIDS?

What about the baby who is always 'asleep upstairs' or 'been taken out for a walk by her Gran' when the midwife asks to see her? The midwife says that she will need to weigh the baby tomorrow and when she arrives with scales the next day no one answers the door. In each of these cases the midwife's supervisor of midwives should be informed. She may be able to help, and at least it is another midwife to share a problem with confidentially.

ROLE OF A SUPERVISOR OF MIDWIVES

A supervisor of midwives can be contacted at all times (there has to be one available 24 hours a day) and she should see herself as a 'guide, counsellor and friend' to the midwives in her area. She is responsible for giving the midwives in her area any information they may need to enable them to function effectively, and she is there to support and promote our profession. Many supervisors give much support to the midwives they are responsible for:

- They give honorary contracts to independent midwives so that they can carry on caring for women they feel would be better off transferred to hospital.
- They ensure that study days in their hospital are well advertised.
- They support and cherish midwives who are supporting women going against medical advice with all the attendant anxieties.
- They listen to midwives and discuss practice in an open way, not substituting their own clinical judgement, but respecting the clinical expertise of the clinician and referring to her and respecting and listening to her decisions.

Supervision is a difficult role, especially for those supervisors who are also managers and whose managerial role involves working in a different way. Supervision at its best is a role that we are not used to. We who are so used to criticising each other and more often say 'Tut, tut' are slowly and with some difficulty learning to say 'Well done, I support you in your struggle for our profession and for women.'

References

HMSO (1979). *Nurses, Midwives and Health Visitors Act 1979.*

Midwives' Information and Resource Services, Westminster Hospital, Dean Ryle St, London SW1 2AP.

Register of Cases I and *II*. Available from Hymns Ancient and Modern Ltd, St Mary's Works, St Mary's Plain, Norwich, Norfolk NR3 3BH.

UKCC. (1986). *Handbook of Midwives' Rules.* United Kingdom Central Council for Nursing, Midwifery and Health Visiting, 23 Portland Place, London W1N 3AF. Tel: 01 637 7181.

UKCC. (1986). *A Midwife's Code of Practice.* United Kingdom Central Council for Nursing, Midwifery and Health Visiting.

Chapter Ten

Special Challenges

Emergencies happen throughout life and we cope with them. Emergencies can occur during pregnancy, labour and the puerperium, and if you have an emergency situation it is highly likely that you will react appropriately. Usually you will find yourself going into 'overdrive' and just reacting without being conscious of thinking your actions through. This is (as far as we can see) the *only* advantage gained from our rather dogmatic type of educational system.

What sort of emergency will the midwife working in the community encounter? And how should she deal with them? A case history (with names changed) may illustrate the midwife's role in an emergency situation.

DURING PREGNANCY

Midwife Claudine is called to Kamla Yadav who is 39 weeks pregnant and having pain. She may be in established labour. Midwife Claudine observes Kamla as she greets her. Kamla's English is very limited and her husband is translating for her. Kamla has been having a pain and indicates that the pain is at the top of her abdomen and is very sharp. Claudine realises that this pain is not coming and going and it is in the wrong place for contractions. During examination Claudine discovers that Kamla has oedematous ankles and a blood pressure of 160/110. Kamla has severe pre-eclampsia, and is having epigastric pain. Claudine has come upon an emergency situation. She needs to telephone for the obstetric flying squad because the epigastric pain may be a sign of impending eclampsia. Claudine already knows which hospital the flying squad comes out from so she telephones the labour ward and alerts them to what is happening so that they can be sure that they bring sedatives with them. If she asks Kamla to pass urine she should keep the whole specimen if there is a suitable container available. It is likely that the urine will be full of albumin and that Kamla will only pass a small amount because her kidneys will be failing.

Claudine telephones Kamla's GP and asks him to come round very quickly with some anti-hypertensive drugs. While they are awaiting the arrival of the flying squad, Claudine makes sure that Kamla is lying quietly and that the curtains are drawn to ensure that the room is as dark as possible. She explains to Kamla and her husband what is happening – that Kamla's blood pressure has gone very high, that she could have a fit if it goes on getting higher, and that she wants Kamla to keep her blood pressure down by relaxing. She speaks in a soothing tone, reassuring her that drugs to bring down her blood pressure are on their way, and leads Kamla through relaxation throughout her body. She tells Kamla's husband that Kamla is not in labour but she might have to have a caesarean section when they get to the hospital or within a few hours.

When people are shocked – which Kamla and her husband will be because 15 minutes ago they were a peaceful couple just wondering if she might be in labour and now they are awaiting the flying squad, and in a short time they will be in hospital and plunged into an alien environment with strange and painful things happening to Kamla – it is difficult for them to take in what you are saying, so it is worth saying what you need to say several times, while they are still in the peace of their own home. Claudine gets Kamla's husband Ravi to explain what is going on to Kamla and she also gets him to gather together a towel, soap, nightdress and comb for Kamla – or just to gather up Kamla's suitcase if she has packed one.

Claudine welcomes the flying squad in a friendly way so that Kamla and Ravi see that Claudine has confidence in these strangers. Kamla will need to be sedated, given anti-hypertensive drugs, transferred to hospital, perhaps given a caesarean section very soon after admission and kept under intensive supervision and care for several days following delivery. If Claudine has documented Kamla's blood pressure, temperature, pulse, oedema, epigastric pain, the size of her uterus, how the baby is lying and the fetal heart rate it will be very useful for the admitting staff to have a base line and history.

BLEEDING IN PREGNANCY

If you are called to a woman who is bleeding during pregnancy, lie her down, keep her still and call her GP. If he is not available telephone the obstetric registrar at the local hospital. If the bleeding is heavy, such as with placenta praevia or with a revealed abruptio placenta, put a towel or several maternity pads between her legs and wrap her in a towel. If the bleeding is concealed she will be showing signs of shock and pain.

Take the woman's pulse frequently (about every five minutes) and her blood pressure. As with all haemorrhage her pulse will become weak and thready and her blood pressure will fall. She needs urgent transfer to hospital either by ordinary ambulance or preferably with the obstetric flying squad. If you carry intravenous equipment it is a good idea to put up a drip and give her some Haemaccel or some other blood volume replacement. Do not put up saline or any other diluting agent as this will aggravate clotting difficulties. It is an emergency situation, so that it is permissible for you to take extraordinary measures. Rule 40 (2) states: 'A practising midwife must not *except in an emergency* undertake any treatment which she has not been trained to give either before or after registration as a midwife and which is outside her sphere of practice.' This is an emergency – your duty is to keep the woman as safe as possible and to keep a record of what you are doing and what is happening, even if you only have a sheet of paper out of your diary: 'A practising midwife shall keep as contemporaneously *as is reasonable* detailed records of observations, care given and medicine or other forms of pain relief administered by her to all mothers and babies' (Rule 42 (1)).

While waiting for the obstetric flying squad the midwife needs to calm the woman, but also to ensure that she knows how serious her condition is – especially for her baby. It is not kind to reassure and to tell her that everything will be all right because it is likely that it won't.

If the woman is only bleeding slightly do not be lulled into a false sense of security – she may start to bleed more heavily at any time. It is essential that she is transferred to hospital and that she is lying down whilst she is being transferred.

EMERGENCIES DURING LABOUR

A couple of case histories may illustrate some useful lessons.

Fiona is booked for a home birth, she has everything ready for the birth and is 39 weeks pregnant. She already has a four-year-old son. Her husband Rick calls midwife Claire at five o'clock in the morning to say that she is in strong labour. When Claire knocks on Fiona's door shortly afterwards she hears the unmistakable sounds of a woman in the second stage of labour, and when Rick opens the door he says, excitedly, 'I think it's coming.'

Claire quickly washes her hands and then crouches down to see whether she can see any signs of full dilatation. She can see signs of full dilatation but at first she cannot make out what she is seeing emerge. It could be a very bald baby, but what is that brown stuff? It's fresh meconium. Fiona is delivering a breech baby. Claire quickly thinks about the baby when it emerges. It may well be shocked and in need of resuscitation. On the other hand the labour is going so smoothly it is highly likely that the baby will come out in excellent condition, but she asks Rick to telephone the GP quickly and to tell him that Fiona is in labour and having a breech birth and the midwife says can he come straight away please. Claire also at the same time gets her resuscitation equipment all ready. She has her notes, or at least a piece of paper, for writing down the times of what is going on. She gets Fiona to stand up with her legs wide apart to increase Fiona's pelvic diameters. Claire has never seen a breech born in any other way than with the woman in lithotomy so she is frightened,

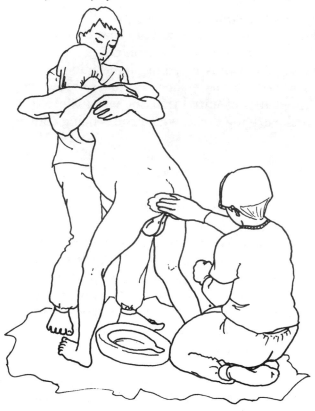

but she needs to reassure herself that until twenty years ago midwives delivered breech babies of multiparous women at home as a normal procedure and that the greatest danger to the baby coming by the breech is that of interference – pulling on the baby and so extending the arms or the head. With the woman standing up the uterus contracts around the baby's head and keeps the head flexed, and by keeping Fiona standing up she is increasing her pelvic diameters. Claire also tries to listen to the fetal heart, and gets herself some sterile gloves ready. When Rick comes back into the room she gets Fiona to cling to him so that when she has a contraction she can drop down and increase her pelvic diameters even more. Claire also equips herself with a warmed towel ready for the baby when it has emerged.

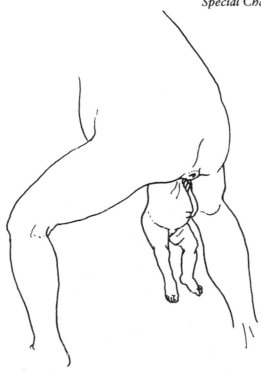

The baby's bottom progresses. Claire sits on the floor behind Fiona. The emerging baby looks strange because what she is looking at is the back of two little legs, or maybe a rather blue foot. Claire warns Fiona that the baby's legs are going to drop down soon which will feel peculiar and tickly. When they do Claire supports them gently and then lets them hang. She may need to press gently behind the knee joint if the baby's legs are extended and if this is splinting the baby's body too much, but usually just leaving the baby alone at all times is the best policy.

The body emerges gradually. Every time a contraction comes Fiona squats down holding on to Rick. Once the umbilicus has descended Claire tries very gently to free a loop of cord so that it isn't pulled, but she is aware that if she is not gentle with the cord it will go into spasm. The baby hangs from the vagina, more and more of its body emerging with

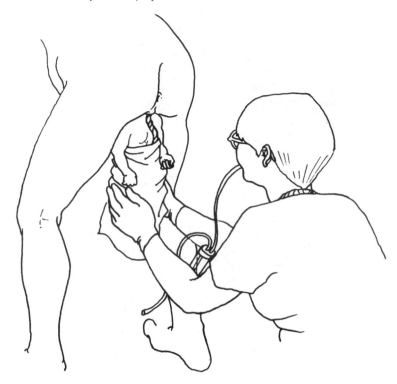

each contraction. Claire keeps the baby as warm as possible by wrapping the warmed towel around her little body. She has also warned Fiona what she wants her to do once the baby is completely hanging from the neck down. Once the baby has delivered up to her neck, Rick lets go of Fiona and she lets her whole trunk go forward onto the bed so that her trunk is slanting downwards towards her head; this tilts her pelvis and reveals the baby's nose and mouth. Claire sucks the baby's nose and mouth out while she waits for the rest of the head to emerge. Once the baby's nose and mouth are visible the baby can breathe. Claire gently supports the head as it comes out so that it doesn't emerge too quickly and in an uncontrolled way.

When the baby is born, she could be shocked and need some massaging and a whiff of oxygen but, if she has been delivered gently, she will usually perk up within a couple of minutes.

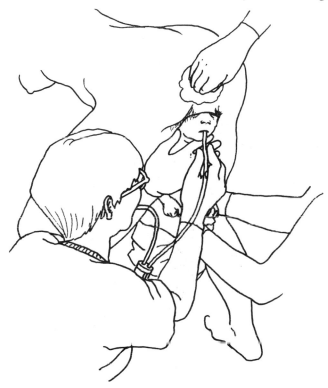

SHOULDER DYSTOCIA

Maggie is with her student Fiona at a home delivery. It is Frances' third baby and she has had two normal deliveries of normal-sized babies. This baby has seemed larger than her first two but no-one is concerned about this as she has always delivered easily before. Frances is in second stage on her hands and knees and pushing gently with each contraction. The baby seems to be taking longer than expected to emerge but the fetal heart is fine when Maggie manages to find it (upside down) with the Sonicaid. Fiona has her sterile gloves on and is ready to deliver. Out comes the crown, the forehead, eyes, nose, mouth and, with some help, the chin – the baby's head is a very big one and the face looks really squashed. The head is only just out and none of the baby's

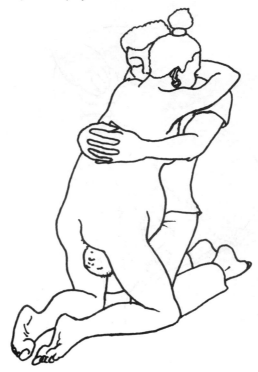

neck can be seen as the mother's body is tight around the baby's neck and it is very difficult for Fiona to feel for the cord.

With the next contraction nothing happens, the baby does not progress out of its mother – the shoulders are not rotating. They are obviously big and have got themselves jammed within the pelvis, Maggie realises that she must get Frances to move her pelvis to free the baby's shoulders. She encourages and helps Frances to get up, first on one foot then on the other, Frances stands up with her knees as wide apart as possible. The action of moving her pelvis frees the baby's shoulders and with the next contraction and quite a bit of traction from Fiona, baby Sarah is born. Sarah is a bit shocked but is a good colour and very soon breathes and starts to cry loudly. She weighs nearly 10 lb when the midwives weigh her.

With shoulder dystocia the need is to move the pelvis so

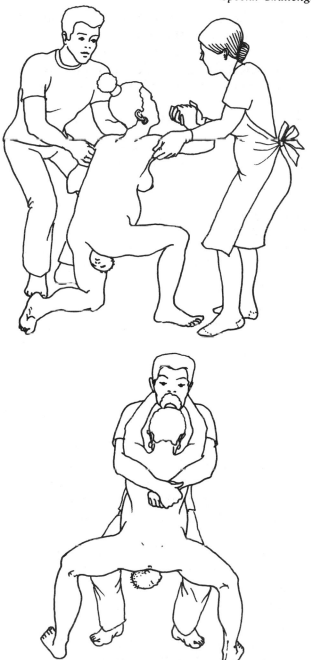

that the baby's shoulders are encouraged to rotate. It probably doesn't matter how the pelvis is rotated – from lying down, to hands and knees; from kneeling to standing up; from standing up to being on all fours – but it is important for the movement to include a tilting of the pelvis.

MECONIUM-STAINED LIQUOR

Often in first labours the baby passes meconium. According to Stirrat, meconium is present in 15% of all deliveries and up to 40% when pregnancy is past term. This can be the greeny colour of stale meconium, which means that the baby experienced some stress within the past few days, or it can be the thick brown of dilute fresh meconium. If during a home birth the woman begins to drain this thick sticky meconium in the liquor, it is best to transfer her to hospital so that the baby can be aspirated and resuscitated by a paediatrician. If the liquor is only stained with stale meconium and the fetal heart is fine, it may be all right to carry on with delivering at home, but the woman needs to be shown how you want her to deliver, so that she is in a position in second stage in which you can aspirate the baby's mouth and larynx before the chest has expanded to take a breath.

The simplest way of aspirating a baby which has had meconium-stained liquor is for the woman to be standing with her back to you, knees bent in a semi-squat, or for the woman to be on all fours as she is delivering. When the baby emerges from the woman in this position the baby's face is towards the midwife and she can then suck out thoroughly the back of the mouth and the larynx. It is possible in this position to remove every bit of meconium before the baby is fully born and wanting to take a breath, especially if the woman refrains from pushing and just pants during a contraction. Carson, Losey et al, all suggest that this method significantly decreases the incidence of meconium aspiration.

CORD PROLAPSE

Cord prolapse is extremely rare and may happen following

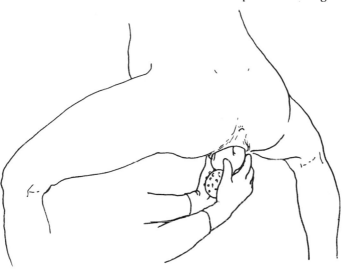

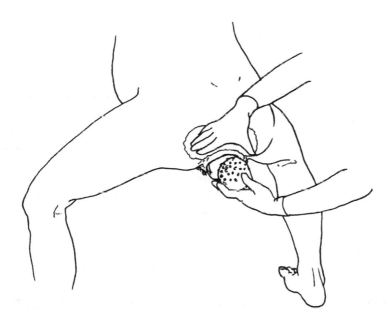

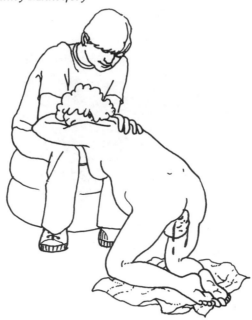

intervention such as artificial rupture of the membranes when the baby's head is not engaged. The possibility of it happening if ever the membranes rupture and the head is not engaged should also be borne in mind. On vaginal examination you will feel something unusual which is pulsating, firm and springy. You may experience a feeling of shock and try to deny that this is what you are feeling. You need to take pressure off the cord to enable the baby to continue to be oxygenated and to transfer the woman as quickly as possible to a maternity unit where she can have a caesarean section virtually on arrival.

In order to take pressure off the cord, the woman must be helped into a knee-chest position with her knees elevated by being on a couple of pillows, and her bottom in the air. Your sterile gloved hand should be inside her vagina pushing the baby's head away from the cord, whilst the obstetric flying squad speeds towards you. The woman will need to be transferred in this same position so she will need to be covered with a blanket so that she is afforded some privacy as she is carried out to the ambulance. Your arm will ache and the woman will also find it very tiring being in this position – soothing words will help you and her through.

POSTPARTUM HAEMORRHAGE

One of the most frightening experiences that a midwife can experience at home is that of postpastum haemorrhage.

The baby is safely delivered, he lies cradled in his mother's arms. She and her husband are cooing at him and he is looking around him with fascination at the world he has joined. They are all awaiting the emergence of the placenta and then the midwife glances down into the bedpan that the woman is sitting on and sees that it is full of blood. The midwife immediately gives the woman an intravenous injection of Syntometrine warning her first, but if the midwife is feeling shocked it may be more sensible for her to give the injection intramuscularly which is undoubtedly easier.

The important thing to do is to deliver the placenta in order to allow the uterus to contract down and stop the bleeding. The placenta is probably lying in the lower uterine segment and stopping the whole uterus from contracting, which is why so much blood is being lost before the delivery of the placenta. Once the injection has been given the midwife needs to help the mother to lie down so that she can palpate her uterus. If it is well contracted she can deliver the placenta by controlled cord traction.

The midwife needs to keep a good check on the uterus after the placenta has delivered to make sure that it remains contracted. She also needs to check the mother's pulse and blood pressure.

If the mother is shocked she should telephone for the doctor, c.f. Rule 40: 'In any case where there is an emergency or where she detects in the health of a mother and baby a deviation from the norm a practising midwife shall call to her assistance a registered medical practitioner, and shall forthwith report the matter to the local supervising authority.'

This could be the GP, but if he is not supportive of birth at home or if he has no specific obstetric qualifications, this might not be helpful. The midwife can ring for the obstetric flying squad. But if the woman's condition doesn't appear to be serious enough to warrant that, the midwife can ring the obstetric registrar on call at the local maternity unit to tell him that she will be bringing the mother in by ambulance.

If bleeding is controlled by delivering the placenta, the uterus stays well contracted and the woman's pulse is strong and regular, with her blood pressure not abnormally low, then there may be no necessity to transfer her to hospital and the midwife may decide to stay with her for a couple of hours to observe her condition. Following that she may suggest steps to counteract probable anaemia: double iron tablets, herbal iron compounds, raisins, molasses, Guinness or Mackeson daily, eggs, chocolate and other iron rich foods.

If the midwife decides to keep the woman at home she still needs to inform a doctor, according to the Midwives' Rules, because there has been a deviation from the norm. It would seem sensible to inform the GP if it is during the daytime, but if it is in the middle of the night it seems ridiculous to wake up the obstetric registrar at the hospital to tell him that you have had a postpartum haemorrhage at home; that you are not bringing the woman in, and you have woken him up specially to make him anxious and to confirm all his worst fears that home births are dangerous and midwives are mad. Probably the best person to contact in this case, in order to help you comply with the Rules, is the supervisor of midwives. Many community midwives keep to hand the telephone number of a sympathetic GP that they can ring about any woman in their area in order to comply with the Rules.

In a couple of days the midwife takes a blood sample to see what the haemoglobin level is, and whether the reticulocyte count is raised because the body is replacing red blood cells as quickly as it can. Once the haemodilution of pregnancy disappears during the first few days after the birth, the haemoglobin rises automatically and the woman who looked ghastly with a haemoglobin of 6 g on Wednesday can look and feel much brighter by the following Tuesday with a haemoglobin of 10 g, especially if she eats iron rich foods.

THE JAUNDICED BABY

Jaundice which the baby is born with or which occurs within the first 36 hours of birth is not normal or physiological and needs urgent action, even if the baby appears otherwise well and is feeding well. The baby probably has a rhesus incompatibility, AB-O incompatibility, an infection, hepatitis or some other liver problem. The baby needs to be seen by a paediatrician before its problems become overwhelming.

Jaundice occurring after 36 hours is usually physiological and can be treated with an increase in light as described in Chapter 6. The increase in light can be tested with the light meter in a camera. The baby's bilirubin level can be tested with a heel prick blood test and it can be seen if the baby has bilirubinuria by testing a wet nappy with a multistix. In *Textbook of Neonatology*, N. R. C. Roberton says, 'There is absolutely no evidence that there is any need to give phototherapy for this condition in infants greater than 37 weeks gestation and 3 kg birthweight until the bilirubin reaches at least 400 µmol/litre (Lewis *et al.*, 1982). Yet this treatment is widely, and therefore in my view completely unjustifiably, administered to enormous numbers of such mildly jaundiced babies per annum in the United Kingdom.'

CHILD ABUSE

Every mother should normally be pleased and proud to show you her lovely baby. If for some reason the baby is 'out' or 'asleep' or otherwise not available to be seen, bells should ring in your head and you should make sure that you see the baby the next day. If you announce your intention of seeing the baby the next day, you may find no reply to your knock when you arrive. In your health district there will be a named person who you must contact in the case of suspected child abuse. You should also inform your supervisor of midwives.

In some families some or all of the children are already on the 'at risk' register. You may need to use all your skills to support the parents in their care of their baby. They will often be parents who have lacked loving parenting themselves. Here the mothering role of the midwife can be extremely useful, if the midwife can see herself as a loving granny or auntie to this family – praising and encouraging the parents and supporting them in their care of their children.

The use of a 'Homestart' scheme could also be looked into. These schemes consist of volunteers taking on the role of 'Auntie' to a family, and the benefits are. very great to families with a high level of deprivation. The interest and support of their 'Auntie' figure helps in many situations where before they felt isolated and defensive. The community midwifery service in conjunction with the Health Visitors, could initiate the setting up of such a scheme to the benefit of the community they serve.

This list of emergencies is of course not exhaustive: we have detailed a few of these very rare occurrences and we hope that we have shown you that YOU CAN COPE, that you are competent and able, well trained and able to provide the sort of care which women need and want – safely, gently and sensitively.

References

Carson, B. S., Losey, R. W., Bowes, W. A., Simmons, M. A. (1976). Combined obstetric and p approach to prevent meconium aspiration syndrome. *American Journal of Obstetrics and Gynecology*. **126**, 6, pp. 712–15

Roberton, N. R. C. (1986). *Textbook of Neonatology*. Edinburgh and London: Churchill Livingstone.

Stirrat, G. M. (1986). *Obstetrics—Pocket Consultant*. Oxford, London, Edinburgh: Blackwell Scientific Publications.

UKCC. (1986). *Handbook of Midwives' Rules*. United Kingdom Central Council for Nursing, Midwifery and Health Visiting, 23 Portland Place, London W1N 3AF. Tel: 01 637 7181.

UKCC. (1986). *A Midwife's Code of Practice*. United Kingdom Central Council for Nursing, Midwifery and Health Visiting.

Chapter Eleven

Caseloads

The new community midwife is presented with a list of names which looks something like this:

Mrs Brown, 35 Ede Way – 7 days
Sharon Coker, 118 Verney Park Road – 5 days
Mrs Russell, 136 Mayhurst Rise – 11 days – sticky eyes
Mrs Hamilton, 69 Owlett Mead – 8 days (gravida 7, fundus slow to involute)
Mrs Lushan, 6 Foxbert Road – 3 days – perineum very swollen
Mrs Rahim, 12 Willard Way – 4 days – sore nipples
Mrs Mugbeh, 49 Upper Farrant St – 2 days
Mrs Belhosa, 88 World's End Road – 6 days
Maggie Chester, 92 Mayhurst Rise – 14 days fundus check
Mrs MacDonald, 118 Sinka St – 9 days (SB baby boy)
Mrs Rajeswaren, 174 Amerton Road – 3 days
Mrs Francis, 2 The Reeves, Sankley Road – AN for booking

A list of twelve women who have been through a huge and life-changing experience, who each have a different story to tell, who each live in very different homes and situations. You have the minimum of information about each woman: you don't even know her first name, whether this is her first baby or her third, whether her labour was traumatic or normal. It is likely that her notes will be inside her home so that when you get there you can read up on what you need to know, but how do you go about visiting them in any sort of order? Where should you begin?

Mrs Mugbeh's baby is only two days old, it would probably be best to start with Mrs Mugbeh in Upper Farrant Street, because she will probably welcome some help with topping and tailing the baby ready for the day. On the other hand, Upper Farrant Street may be the other side of the district from where you live and this may be Mrs Mugbeh's third baby and she is managing very well without you arriving at her door very early in the morning. If Upper Farrant Street is the other side of the district from your base, the rush-hour congestion may make it simpler for you to visit women who are near you first in the mornings.

With only a few visits to make and in a rural community it would seem sensible to see women in date order, leaving the oldest babies and mothers until last. With a large number of mothers and babies to fit in it is often a matter of where women live. A map of the area is an essential piece of equipment, plus several highlighter pens of varying colours. Sit down first thing in the morning before you start and highlight Ede Way, Verney Park Road, Mayhurst Rise, Owlett Mead, Foxbert Road, Willard Way, Upper Farrant Street, World's End Road, Mayhurst Rise, Sinka Street, Amerton Road and Sankley Road. You have noted that you have two visits in Mayhurst Rise so obviously it would seem sensible to do those two visits after each other. Having highlighted the roads you will have them in your map for future reference and when in a few weeks someone gives you a woman to visit in Owlett Mead, you will remember the name and it will be easier to find.

Each day mark the roads you are going to in highlighter pen. If you start with yellow, you can then go onto pink, then red, then green and progressing to darker and darker colours so that you won't have to replace your map for some time. Another way of identifying where you are going is to pin your map to a large pinboard or soft wooden board and buy some coloured map pins from a stationers. Stick a map pin into each road you need to visit and take them out when the visit has been made.

Having highlighted the roads you will then probably be able to see a logical sequence for your visits and hopefully find somewhere in the middle to have some lunch. Many community midwives end up having their lunch in the car, some seek the haven of a local health centre which may have a staff sitting-room, some go to the maternity hospital and use the staff canteen, some go to a local municipal building, some go home. If you have a student midwife with you, she may not have brought a packed lunch and, even though she can buy some sandwiches, it may be somewhat claustrophobic for you both to be closeted in your car when she is dying to find a phone to telephone her sister to ask her something important. It can often be a tricky problem, especially in sleazy areas. Often the best lunches are found in pubs, but if you are decked out in your uniform it hardly seems appropriate to go to the local pub for a bite. You feel immensely conspicuous in your uniform and can be the butt of all sorts of advances: 'Are you a girl guide, Miss? – because I've lost my purse and haven't got no bus fare. Could you let me have 50 pence to get home?' Or, on entering the pub: 'Cor, look here lads, here's the nurses. Stan here's got a headache, Miss. Can you come and soothe 'is brow?'

There are often obvious priorities. Mrs Belhosa may tell you that tomorrow she has to take her elder son to the out-patient department so could you please visit her early in the morning. Mrs Rahim may have very sore nipples and you want to visit her as soon as possible in the morning tomorrow to see if they are any better.

Mrs Reeves, who is antenatal and needs a booking history done, may not be expecting you and may be at work. Is it possible to get a phone number so that you can telephone her for arranging an approximate time? With 12 visits and each visit taking a minimum time of 25 minutes and with Mrs MacDonald, whose baby was stillborn, likely to take longer because of her probable need to talk, you need to calculate travelling time as well as just the visit. So some of these visits will need to be done in the afternoon, but if you leave Mrs Chester until the afternoon will she still be in when you get there?

Until you get to know your area and until you get to know the women, it is a case of just doing your best and hoping that it will come out as right as possible.

One of the factors that those visited complain about most

is the unpredictability of our visits: 'You never knew what time she was coming, and then when she did come it was always just as you'd got the baby to sleep and she wanted to look at him.' Our visits can be stressful for the new parents but also they can be a source of intense pleasure.

With all the women's names and addresses in your diary a good way to put them in the order that you have decided to visit is to have a coloured felt-tip pen and number each name and address. It is also a good idea to write your mileometer reading at the top of the page when you get in the car in the morning, and again in the evening when you finish.

In some districts midwives are required to fill in highly complicated time sheets and statistics. It is often an idea to keep these in the car on a clip board and to fill them up each day when you park outside your own home – likewise *Register of Cases I* which you may be required to fill in. These charts can be very difficult to read, with little tiny squares over a space of 31 days. Highlighter pens can be useful here too. If you highlight the weekends, or every third day, so that you have a point of reference in this sea of little squares it can make the filling in much simpler.

HOW MANY CASES?

It is difficult to decide what is too heavy a caseload for a community midwife because it is easy to just go on and on doing postnatal visits. But it is highly likely that the community midwife of the future will, like her predecessor of the 1930s and 40s, be undertaking the total care of pregnant women – not in isolation, as midwives have in the last few decades, but working in a team or group practice of midwives. How do we decide how many cases a year is a reasonable caseload per midwife?

In the 1940s the Central Midwives Board made an attempt to give guidance to domiciliary midwives and stated that 72 cases *per annum* was the maximum that should be cared for by a midwife. This was both to protect the municipal midwife from being required to undertake too much by her employers, and to protect the public from private midwives who were overbooking in an attempt to make ends meet.

Midwives in independent practice today appear to book about 24 to 30 pregnant women a year, if they are practising single-handed, but say that this can be safely increased if they are working in partnership with others.

It would appear that there are at present no guidelines to assist health authorities in determining how many midwives. This is something that the midwifery profession needs to address.

Mary worked in the late 1950s in domiciliary practice as an employee of a county council, having one day off a week and one weekend off a month. She says that she has *no wish* to return to this! She feels that perhaps something in the order of 40 cases per midwife per annum would allow a satisfactory level of care and a satisfactory off-duty for midwives working in groups. This is only a suggestion, and different districts would need to adjust this upwards or downwards depending on the type of area. A stable indigenous population in a prosperous semi-rural area may enable the midwife to have a higher caseload, while an area with difficult social problems and high-risk mothers may require lower caseloads as health visitor colleagues have found. On the other hand a widespread rural area, whilst not having the problems of the inner cities, poses problems of long distances to be travelled and the problems of loneliness and isolation. Maybe a lower caseload will be appropriate in these areas.

On the subject of caseloads – if midwives feel that their caseload is so great that they are unable to provide care of a high enough standard, there are several measures they may take. The problem, of course, is that they all take time, and when a midwife is very overloaded this is the very time when she 'hasn't enough time' to do something about her workload. The *Code of Professional Conduct for the Nurse, Midwife and Health Visitor* published by the UKCC in November 1984 states: 'Every registered nurse, midwife and health visitor is accountable for his or her practice, and in the

exercise of professional accountability shall ... have regard
to the workload of and the pressures on professional colleagues and subordinates and take appropriate action if these
are seen to be such as to constitute abuse of the individual
practitioner and/or to jeopardise safe standards of practice'
(Paragraph 11).

What this means of course is that it is *you* who are
responsible for *your* practice, and if you have too heavy a
workload it is *your* responsibility to bring it down to a safe
and acceptable level. It also means that your managers are
responsible for ensuring that your workload should not constitute abuse of the individual practitioner and/or jeopardise
safe standards of practice. But no manager can know that
you are overworked unless you tell her. If you just grumble
about being 'overworked and underpaid' she will take it that
you are just grumbling, and that she can ignore your grum-
bles because what you are doing is just letting off steam and
having a good moan.

It is also your professional duty to 'make known to appropriate persons or authorities any circumstances which could
place patients/clients in jeopardy or which militate against
safe standards of practice' (Paragraph 10).

So let us imagine that you, after careful consideration,
have decided that you have too heavy a caseload. A surfeit
once every now and then probably cannot be helped, but you
are finding that every day you are rushing round and are
unable to provide the sort of care you would expect to be
able to provide to women having babies. You first of all need
to have sorted out in your mind what you consider to be a
standard of good practice and, if possible, have detailed that
right at the beginning of your appointment so that you can
refer to what you thought you should be doing when you
first started this job.

If you feel that your are being so overloaded that you cannot provide a safe standard of practice you should inform
your manager. You can do this verbally at first but you need
to keep a record of doing it – in your diary. Your manager
may not do anything about it (and, you are quite right, often

it seems that she *cannot* do anything about it and that you are just increasing her burden by worrying her). However, this charitable reasoning on your part will not help you when you are before the professional conduct committee having made an error because you were so overworked, nor will it help the woman you have neglected or made a mistake over, or the parents of the baby who has died as a result. Having told your manager that your workload is such that you cannot provide an adequate safe standard of care, you need to write to her (keeping a copy of the letter) and you need to discuss the problem with your supervisor of midwives. This may be one and the same person or there may be another supervisor of midwives you can go to. Tell her that you wish to see her as your supervisor of midwives, as your 'guide, counsellor and friend' and, as such, it is she who sets standards of practice within her area. If she is unable to help, your next step can be to write to your local supervising authority – in the United Kingdom this is usually your regional health authority, and the responsibility is taken by the regional nursing officer with help from the regional legal adviser. Tell them that you feel that your workload is so great that you are unable to provide care of a safe and satisfactory standard; send a copy of the letter to your local supervisor of midwives and engage the help of your local steward of the Royal College of Midwives, your professional organisation or health service trade union. Often you will feel very alone while doing all this. Midwives are often very lazy at doing anything for themselves, probably because they feel overworked, tired, depressed and impotent. Even if all your colleagues are being equally overworked, they will probably leave all the action to you. You will need supportive relationships to strengthen you: the Association of Radical Midwives, your local Royal College of Midwives branch, the local National Childbirth Trust or AIMS, the mothers you have looked after during the past couple of years – all these people are as interested as you are in the provision of a good service for women.

You should also try and galvanise your local branch of the

Royal College of Midwives into action. As members of the work force you could all be finding out:

- The midwifery establishment over the past two years and the actual numbers of midwives employed – has it varied at all?
- The numbers of women being cared for over the past two years – have they varied at all? What about the number of antenatal visits, visits in order to carry out a home assessment, length of stay, postnatal visits, deliveries, have these increased in the last two years?
- Look at the numbers of community midwives – has their number increased/decreased in the past two years?
- What about the community midwives' workload? Are they being expected to do more? More postnatal visits? More bookings at home?

If the number of women being treated in any way goes up – so should the number of midwives.

List those duties which midwives are doing which are not midwifery duties, such as cleaning floors when in the labour ward, taking specimens to the laboratory; and those duties which properly belong to a midwife which someone else is doing – a ready example is postnatal care given to mothers and babies by staff other than midwives. In the Midwife's Code of Practice, Paragraph 5 'Arranging for a Substitute', reads:

> 'A person other than a registered midwife or a registered medical practitioner shall not attend a woman in childbirth.'
> 'A midwife or an employing authority should not arrange for anyone to act as the substitute for a midwife other than another registered midwife eligible to practise or a registered medical practitioner.'

Under 'The Activities of a Midwife' her role is defined as:

> 'She must be able to give the necessary supervision, care and advice to women during pregnancy, labour and the postpartum period, to conduct deliveries on her own responsibility and to care for the newborn and the infant.'

Again in 'The Activities of a Midwife' we read that she is expected:

> 'To care for and monitor the progress of the mother in the post-natal period and to give all necessary advice to the mother on infant care to enable her to ensure the optimum progress of the new-born infant.'

Thus if someone other than a midwife is performing post-natal care this is contrary to the Midwife's Code of Practice. The midwife needs to ensure that it is she who is performing postnatal care on women and their babies – not anyone else. If you are aware that you are not able to give the appropriate quality of care to mothers and babies all the midwives (or as many as you can muster) need to write a joint letter to state to your managers that you can no longer be accountable for the care of the mothers and babies because of the unsafe staffing levels (quoting the details of the information that you have gathered). It is a hard action to take, but it is *you* who are responsible for safe care for the mothers and babies you are caring for.

If still nothing is being done about the workload, you should write to the investigating officer at your National Board (address on p. 179) and state that you wish to allege that your manager or supervisor has contravened paragraph 11 of the *Code of Professional Conduct for Nurses, Midwives and Health Visitors* and that the workload which she is allocating to you is such that it constitutes abuse of the individual practitioner and jeopardises safe standards of care. With the letter send copies of any correspondence and the details of the instances when you have verbally informed your manager of the 'circumstances which could place patients/clients in jeopardy or which mitigate against safe standards of practice' (Paragraph 10).

Eventually the establishment will be increased and vacancies will be filled, if you hold out for better care for women. We have created a terrible system, a hierarchy in which those who are actually caring for the women and their babies are at the bottom of the heap where they are expected to have no opinions or ideas of their own. These are expected to come from above, but this is a nonsense because usually ideas come from the workplace. You need to be thinking whether you are actually doing midwifery and whether your skills could be better deployed and someone else employed to do the jobs that you are doing which do not need to be done by a qualified midwife. Which of these jobs needs a qualified midwife?

Chaperoning a doctor. *No.*
Conducting an antenatal consultation. *Yes.*
Scrubbing for a caesarean section. *Probably.*
Cleaning the labour ward floor. *No.*
Making a bed. *Not usually.*
Bathing and checking a baby. *Yes.*
Supervising breastfeeding. *Yes.*
An artificial feed mixing demonstration. *Yes.*
Filling in a form. *Depends on the form.*
Applying an ice pack to a woman's sore perineum. *Yes.*

If your unit is short of midwives is there a crèche? Job-sharing? Room for part-time midwives? An opening for midwives truly to practise fully as midwives so that they are more ready to return to practice?

You and *I, we* – the midwives on the job – are responsible for the service provided. Make sure the managers hear what you have to say. Set up opportunities for discussions and swapping of ideas and remember how isolated managers often feel and that they need your support and cherishing in the same way that you need theirs. We have to learn to 'manage upwards' as well as expecting others to 'manage downwards'. Support can come in strange ways, like the Board's visits to the School of Midwifery which insists on a bigger midwifery library before the school can be used to train midwives – which means that the midwifery library grows overnight. The threat of being reported to the UKCC for failing to 'have regard to the workload of and the pressures on professional colleagues and subordinates and take appropriate action if these are seen to be such as to constitute abuse of the individual practitioner and/or to jeopardise safe standards of practice' will make miraculous things happen to staffing levels which will almost grow overnight!

References

Register of Cases I and *II*. Available from Hymns Ancient and Modern Ltd, St Mary's Works, St Mary's Plain, Norwich, Norfolk NR3 3BH.

UKCC. (1986). *Handbook of Midwives' Rules*. United Kingdom Central Council for Nursing, Midwifery and Health Visiting, 23 Portland Place, London W1N 3AF. Tel: 01 637 7181.

UKCC. (1984). *A Midwife's Code of Practice*. United Kingdom Central Council for Nursing, Midwifery and Health Visiting.

Chapter Twelve

The Teaching Community Midwife

As midwives working in the community we are often asked to provide experience for student midwives and to teach them about working in the community and how we practise.

This is of course part of our role as practising midwives. Wherever we practise we are teaching, whether it be new or prospective parents, or nurse students undertaking maternity care experience, or new young doctors. During our training we will have had an introduction to teaching skills.

The community midwife who has a student midwife attached to her will need to develop further the teaching role that may only have been touched on during her own training.

The English National Board has identified and responded to this need by developing and offering to midwives Course 997: 'Teaching in Clinical Practice for Midwives'. Hopefully most teaching midwives will be given the opportunity by their employing authority to undertake this course. However, it is not yet mandatory, and there will be many midwives coming into community practice and asked to have a student who have not yet undertaken Course 997. We think that all community midwives required to take students should ask to go on this course. It is a minimum length of fifteen days and can replace a statutory refresher course.

The midwife who has an attached student can gain a great deal from the experience. It is a great responsibility to have a student. One has responsibility to the individual student, to our profession, and of course to the women whom we are attending and whom we ask to agree to the student's presence.

Having a student can also be a great pleasure, and an opportunity for the midwife herself to learn. It is very refreshing and challenging to have a student sitting in the car, following one around, questioning, then undertaking supervised practice, gaining confidence, requiring less supervision, and blossoming as she learns and becomes more experienced. Many of us remember 'our' midwives and the training we received from them. When we think of that experience, whether it had been very good or very bad, we certainly will realise how important it was, and it can make us resolve that we will try to make the community experience of the students entrusted to us as positive and educationally valuable as possible.

A PREPARATORY MEETING BETWEEN MIDWIFE AND STUDENT

It is very helpful to both the student and the midwife if they can meet about a week or so before the student comes out. The midwife should make an appointment to see the student and while the atmosphere should be relaxed and informal, it should also be structured so that both people have the opportunity to get the maximum benefit from it.

When making the appointment to see the student some teaching midwives send a letter of invitation and ask the student to meet them. We should identify that the meeting will cover things like off-duty arrangements, so that if she is likely to have any off-duty requests, or other commitments she can come prepared with dates. We should ask her to try to identify her strengths and weaknesses so that her community experience can be arranged with this in mind.

At the meeting both the midwife and the student should discuss their expectations of each other. The likely hours of work should be clarified, on-call arrangements discussed, transport and communications organised. It is useful for the midwife to find out how much previous experience the student has had of working in a community setting. The student should be encouraged to discuss what she expects to learn, and the midwife should state her aims for the student during the meeting. Together they might set some goals. The mid-

wife should ensure that the student understands the importance of confidentiality when working in people's homes.

HELPING A STUDENT MAKE THE MOST OF HER COMMUNITY EXPERIENCE

In the first few days of working together we should not
expect too much of our students, particularly if the 'community experience' is taking place early in their training. Let
them settle into the community, perhaps just as observers to
start with, but having them participate in the care of mother
and baby as soon as possible remembering that most of us
learn and retain what we have learnt by 'doing' rather than
by just observing.

It is useful to have the student have 'her' cases. Even if she
is very early in her training and needing close supervision, she
will learn by following a case from booking clinic, to home
visit, to any discussions with other professionals, e.g. health
visitor.

Ideally she can be introduced to several women whose
babies are likely to arrive during her time in the community
so that she can study, and get to know, the family antenatally, intranatally, and postnatally.

During visits to the home we will sometimes find it difficult to let the student 'lead' and the temptation to interfere
can be very great, but unless the student is actually doing
something that is frankly dangerous, we should not correct
her in front of the woman, but rather discuss the matter pri-
vately as soon as we leave the home. Sometimes one can in-
tervene tactfully and suggest a more appropriate course of
behaviour. The teaching midwife needs to help the student
develop confidence, but also needs to ensure that that confidence is based on good practice.

During postnatal visits it is a great temptation to say, 'You
do the baby, and I'll do the mum and we'll change over at the
next house.' We must refrain from this. The mother and
baby should be cared for as one unit by the student. It is difficult to observe carefully what the student is doing with the

baby while one is making a proper examination of the mother, and likewise the student will not be able to observe and learn from us if her attention is on the baby. Most important of all, she will fail to have the opportunity to develop *her* teaching and counselling skills by teaching the mother about her baby.

ENCOURAGING A STUDENT TOWARDS INDEPENDENCE AND SELF-RESPONSIBILITY

The student will be anxious to do her best, she will know that we shall be writing a report on her, she will want a good report, she may feel diffident about questioning us or challenging the way we do things. Students from other cultures may be totally unused to questioning a teacher. We cannot hope in the time at our disposal to affect a total change in this attitude but it is up to us to take the lead and reassure her that we shall welcome and encourage her questions. Some of us have come to question our own practices, and have sometimes affected changes in response to penetrative questions from students.

We are the 'role model' for our students. This can be a daunting thought! We may sometimes do things based on our experience, perhaps take shortcuts based on our experience, perhaps not always follow the book. If we do this with a student in attendance we must explain carefully, or expect the student to question. If we do something that is outside the student's experience, and do not explain, and the student does not question, we should ask ourselves why, and raise the subject ourselves.

During her community experience the student may have to arrange to have a day with the health visitor, attend child welfare clinics, family planning clinics, etc. It is up to her to make these arrangements. We should resist the temptation to do it for her and while we would expect her to consult us, we should not take the responsibility from her.

We need to ensure that the student has adequate time for preparation and study, and that she has access to journals and research material relevant to community practice. We should encourage her by our example to be aware of research in midwifery and of the importance of study and keeping up-to-date after qualification and registration.

Most midwife teachers will liaise and consult with the teaching community midwife who has an attached student, but it is our duty to approach them if we encounter any difficulties. Midwife educationalists can give us guidance and encouragement if we find we need help in our teaching role.

Towards the end of her training, the student in the community should be given the opportunity to practise without the close supervision needed in her early training. This will be arranged in a variety of ways depending on different circumstances. If the student has her own transport, or can conveniently do visits by public transport, she can arrange a list for herself, discuss the probable management of each case, and off she goes, reporting back to the teaching midwife. If independent transport cannot be arranged, the situation is more difficult, but she must be enabled to do visits without close supervision even if this means that the midwife sits outside in the car.

It is vitally important that, with the expected increase in home births, the midwife of the future is competent and confident to provide this service. Whenever possible arrangements should be made so that the student has an opportunity to attend any home births that occur during her training. At the end of her training it is ideal if she can undertake the birth alone with the midwife close at hand but not in the room.

The woman's permission must always be sought for the student's attendance. It is useful to mention how grateful the midwife is to the women who permitted her to learn, and of course the woman must be reassured that the student will not be in attendance unless we are confident about her abilities, and that a qualified midwife will always be supervising.

ASSESSING AND SUPPORTING A STUDENT

At our initial meeting we discussed our goals with the student, and our objectives. During her time with us we will be continuously assessing our progress towards achieving them, congratulating her and recognising her increasing competence. If we feel that the student is not making the hoped-for progress we should carefully consider possible reasons for this and possible ways in which we can help her. Are we expecting too much? Are we failing to give her the time to think and consolidate her learning? Has she any personal or private problems? If we are seriously concerned about a student we should discuss the matter with the course tutor and seek to find ways of helping the student to improve.

As the community midwife/student relationship is such a one-to-one situation and therefore fairly intense, there will inevitably be a few occasions when personalities will conflict. As the senior in the relationship it is up to the midwife to try to resolve this, and confront the problem. Sometimes we can overcome the difficulty with honesty and understanding, but occasionally the personality conflict is such that the course tutor should be asked to place the student with another midwife.

It is sad when this happens, and the midwife may have feelings of failure and rejection, as can the student. It can help both if they can seek counselling perhaps from the teacher, or a trusted friend, or from the supervisor of midwives. If a teaching midwife takes over a student from a colleague it can be a very stressful situation which will require very skilful handling, giving the student the opportunity for a fresh start without any criticism of her former teacher. With care it can be made a positive learning experience about personalities, conflicts, and the importance to us all of happy relationships.

At the end of the course an evaluation meeting will be arranged by the school of midwifery. Attendance can be enormously helpful to both the students and the midwives who have taught them. We owe it to our students to make every effort to attend these gatherings, not only because it is usually a very pleasant social occasion with tea and lots of lovely food, but because it is really encouraging to hear our young midwives of the future speaking out and assessing their training, underlining our successes, and pointing to areas where they think we could improve. They are almost invariably right!

Chapter Thirteen

Working Together

HOW CAN I GET TO KNOW YOU WHEN I NEVER SEE YOU?

We are always present for ourselves – we are inside our own bodies and we are always with ourselves. Thus the midwife who works on Ward Six feels that she is always on Ward Six, but in fact for the women on Ward Six that midwife is someone who is here this morning (early shift) and tomorrow evening (late shift) but not the next day or the day after that (days off). Then the women go home, so that midwife was only a tiny part of their experience in Ward Six.

Here's another example. Think warm and loving thoughts about someone you trained with but haven't seen for a while. You have thought about that person, you have devoted time to her, but she doesn't know that. You could devote warm and loving thoughts to her for twenty minutes a week – seventeen hours a year of your time could be devoted to this person and she would never know about it unless you directly communicate with her. Our relationship with everyone is like this. What is important and what matters to other people is how often they see you or how often they hear from you – either by phone or by letter. How often you think about them actually doesn't intrude upon their consciousness and become part of their reality.

It often needs conscious planning to nurture relationships, and a definite commitment. Relationships are incredibly important to us and our feeling of wellbeing, and often we manage somehow to spend hours of our time with people whose relationship with us is very shallow – chatting with a neighbour or a work aquaintance, chatting with a shopkeeper or the milkman, and all this time is being taken away from the people we really care about and relationships we need to nurture.

Take a few moments to list those people that it is important for you to develop a relationship with in order that your work flows smoothly. If you are working in the community we envisage that the list may look something like this:

All the other community midwives
Community senior midwife
Director of midwifery services
GPs in this practice
GPs in the practice down the road
Health visitors
Midwives in the hospital antenatal clinic
Midwives in the labour ward
Secretary/clerk for community midwives
Medical records staff for hospital notes
Consultant obstetricians
Registrars

Then get yourself an exercise book with squared paper. Make a list of your work colleagues down the pages, and then along the top divide the squares into months or weeks and decide how often you are going to make contact with each group. For instance, it is unlikely that you need to make contact with the consultant obstetricians more than once every six weeks – though you may need to see them more often if you are involved in a project with one of them. The midwives in the hospital antenatal clinic might be put down every four or every six weeks; on the other hand you may do a clinic there yourself every week so you will be seeing them every week, so you would put them in your 'Mark Book' as weekly.

Each person's list is totally individual. Some people you will need, or decide, to see more often than others, but if you don't have a systematic way of ensuring that you are seeing or speaking to people, you will find that you rarely see many of them and that your relationship with them will not be as influential or as useful as it needs to be.

For instance, one of us often takes labouring women into the labour ward. When she first started in this area there was a feeling of 'us' in the labour ward and 'them' – the intruders from the community. It was extremely important to improve relationships. Women suffer when they come into a labour ward where the atmosphere is unwelcoming and the midwife feels that she is working despite the system rather than in partnership with it. The problem was solved when the midwife asked if she might eat her packed lunch with the labour ward midwives whenever she was in the vicinity. Sitting there in the staff sitting-room, frequently eating lunch together, formed a bond between the midwives, and now whenever she takes a woman into the hospital, the midwife and her labouring mother are welcomed. The midwife knows every staff member by name, they help her to clear up after the labour if they are not busy, they show her where things are kept when she can't find them. The relationship is warm and supportive, a shared pleasure for both the community midwife and the labour ward midwives, and beneficial to the women.

Another example is the relationship you have with the consultant obstetricians or even the registrars. Often they will support a midwife they know in doing something innovatory but will take fright if the midwife is a total stranger. This can lead to an embarrassing situation when one midwife in a unit is enabled to practise fully as a midwife whilst all the rest are bound down with unit policies and procedures. Often this owes less to the former's skill as a midwife than to her skill as a communicator and her relationships with the doctors. In this day and age, whatever we may think, it is the consultant obstetricians who hold the power in labour wards. If you can build a relationship with them of affection and trust, this can enable you to practise fully. It takes time and effort and can be daunting to take on building a relationship with figures who often seem remote, but this may be the only way to be treated as an equal. Unfortunately there is always a small minority of doctors who are less interested in equal relationships than in being captain of the team. A united stand may be necessary if this individual is preventing you from carrying out good midwifery care. The local Royal College of Midwives or health service trade union branch, the national RCM, the unit midwifery group, the Association of Radical Midwives, AIMS, the Maternity Services Liaison Committee, the local supervising authority, all these bodies and more can be mobilised if women are being deprived of optimum care.

Having listed all your work colleagues according to how often you intend to ensure you contact them, you can then tick off on your squares when you have seen or spoken with them. The contact may be quite casual – meeting each other on the stairs, for instance, and having a chat; seeing one of the registrars in the dining room and joining him for lunch; taking an article that you have found interesting to the director of midwifery services; ringing up your fellow community midwife to ask her how her dog is after its operation; sending a little note of sympathy when you hear that one of the GP's children has broken an arm; taking some apples out of your garden to the clerk; giving the GPs some old magazines for their waiting room; making a point of discussing a family with the health visitors or sharing with them some news about a community project. Often little and seemingly casual actions mean a great deal and bind you to other people with invisible cords – you understand them and how they tick and what is important to them, and they understand you and develop loyalty towards you.

PRESENTING YOUR PROPOSALS AT MEETINGS

The same type of 'homework' needs to be done when a matter which is important to you is to be discussed at a meeting. Don't expect that any idea you have put forward will be taken on just because it is sensible and rational. Any innovation will be threatening to the members of the meeting. If it matters to you, it is essential that you go to every member of the forthcoming meeting and explain the idea fully so that they can see how sensible it is. If you can, go to see the majority of the members of the meeting – or all the members is better, because one or two members can always sway a meeting, though the more you have on your side the better. This takes time, but sometimes it can be combined with your weekly/six-weekly contact with that specific person. It has to be said that in a busy life this can take ages and is annoying, especially when the idea that you want to get agreed at the meeting is eminently sensible. The homework that you do may ensure that you are able to achieve the changes that you want. The other realisation has to be that even if you fail to convince the assembled meeting of the validity of your idea the first time, you should try again in six months' time and then again six months after that (or it could be four monthly). Eventually most of the things that you want to achieve will come to pass, but the patience needed in order for this to happen is enormous.

RELATIONSHIPS WITH USER ORGANISATIONS

Some of the most important people in your life will invariably be members of the women's groups – the women you have delivered/looked after/taught. Some may be members of the National Childbirth Trust, the Association for Improvements in the Maternity Services, the Society to Promote Home Confinements, the Association of Breastfeeding Mothers, the Twins Club and the La Leche League. Make contact with each of the groups active in your area. The NCT will have postnatal support systems and breastfeeding counsellors, their antenatal classes are often an excellent example of adult education at its best. They will be glad to share with you skills and ideas while you can share knowledge and ideas with them.

Many women who are breastfeeding will be really glad to know some other mothers who are breastfeeding or to have a knowledgeable mother's phone number to ring in case of problems and anxieties. The NCT, the Association of Breastfeeding Mothers and the La Leche League all have counsellors and groups of breastfeeding mothers who give support and cherishing to other mothers.

Many of the groups are consulted over maternity service matters, often they have members on the Community Health

Council or on the Maternity Services Liaison Committee. They can be very useful people to lobby about the changes which could be achieved in your health district. You will also find great support from talking with people who care as deeply as you do yourself about how women give birth. The Association for Improvements in the Maternity Services (AIMS) is a more politically aware organisation than the others and it can be extremely useful to have a relationship with AIMS. They can often achieve what you find impossible. For instance, the community midwives in one area found that they were becoming increasingly overwhelmed with postnatal visits, more and more women were being discharged earlier and earlier from hospital so the number of women they were being asked to see grew and grew. As the community midwives became more and more stressed and overworked they approached their senior midwife and pointed out that they could not work like this, that the care they were able to provide to the women was not satisfactory. She retaliated by suggesting that the domino deliveries that they had booked should all be cancelled and carried out by the hospital staff. The community midwives then wrote to their director of midwifery services to point out that this was not satisfactory but they found it difficult to go against their senior midwife. The director of midwifery services then decided that all home confinements should be stopped because the community midwives were too overworked. The community midwives persuaded the women involved to contact AIMS and AIMS were able to pursue the matter with vigour, resulting in an increase in community midwife staffing levels and reinstatement of both domino and home deliveries.

RELATIONSHIPS WITH STATUTORY BODIES

Just because the statutory bodies seem to be a long way away in London doesn't mean that they cannot help the ordinary midwife working away in her district – you are just the person that they want to contact and help. The great beauty of working in a small profession is that every member of it is accessible to each one of us. Both the statutory bodies have a professional officer for midwifery who will be pleased to answer your queries. The National Boards are responsible for education and practice in all midwifery training establishments and the United Kingdom Central Council (UKCC) is responsible for professional conduct. If you have a query or an anxiety about how midwifery is being practised in your area there are several steps you can take to gain support in your anxieties and guidance for action.

The local branch of your professional organisation or trade union should be able to help you. If it isn't a very supportive branch, your local group of the Association of Radical Midwives will be helpful and supportive. Going to one of their national meetings is a good idea especially if you let the secretary know first that you want to discuss a problem so that it will be given space on the agenda. The person who should be your guide, supporter and friend is your supervisor of midwives. If you go to her and say that you wish to speak to her as the supervisor of midwives she should abandon her role as manager (if that is what she is) and talk to you as the supervisor of midwives, and in this role you should both be on the same side. This may be impossible for her to do, so remember that she is acting on behalf of the local supervising authority and you also have access to them. Ring your regional health authority and ask to speak to the regional nursing (*sic*) adviser. Ask her if she is acting as the local supervising authority and if you could discuss a problem to do with midwifery practice in your area. You may find that the regional legal adviser is the person who actually deals with all problems to do with midwifery. They are often helpful because so much of what we do has to do with our Rules (which are the law of the land) and a lawyer can often understand very well.

Another avenue which can be explored is to ring the Royal College of Midwives and ask to speak to the professional officer. She will have unbiased advice to offer.

It is often appreciated by all the people mentioned if you ask them your question and then offer to ring back in five minutes – or ask them to ring you back in five minutes, so that they can put together their thoughts.

The professional officer (midwifery) at the National Board or the professional officer (midwifery) at the UKCC will also be glad to help with any queries you have about your practice or your educational needs. It is important not to feel intimidated and to realise that it is you, as a practitioner who is spearheading your profession, and who the UKCC needs to hear from. In the Nurses, Midwives and Health Visitors Act 1979 Paragraph 2: (5) 'The powers of the Council shall include that of providing, in such manner as it thinks fit, advice for nurses, midwives and health visitors on standards of professional conduct.' Likewise the UKCC's *Code of Professional Conduct for the Nurse, Midwife and Health Visitor* says: 'The Council will welcome suggestions and comments for consideration in (its) periodic review of the Code of Professional Conduct.'

The addresses of the statutory bodies are at the end of this book – use them, the Royal College of Midwives, the Association of Radical Midwives and your local supervising authority as well as your local supervisor as supportive friends – your job is stressful, you need as many supportive friends as you can muster.

WORKING IN A GROUP

In order to provide a greater degree of continuity of care for women having babies midwives are forming themselves into small groups or teams, and taking responsibility for the continuous care of a specific number of women who they are able really to get to know. They provide antenatal, intranatal and postnatal care for the women and in so doing try to provide the type of care that women have been asking us for.

The principles are set out in the Association of Radical Midwives' *The Vision*:

'In 10 years time 60–70% of midwives will work in community based group practices of 2–5 midwives ... These midwives will be responsible for the care of the vast majority of women. ...

30–40% of midwives will be hospital-based, and organised in teams. These teams, working with a consultant obstetrician, will be responsible for the antenatal, intranatal and postnatal care of the 15% of women who present with complications at booking or who develop them during pregnancy.'

And we find the following in the Royal College of Midwives' *The Role and Education of the Future Midwife in the United Kingdom*:

'That the future management and statutory supervision of the midwifery service would be enhanced by a team approach to care. This should be reflected across the service within any health authority, and midwives should be peripatetic and competent to practice within the community or hospital environment with equal ease. Such mobility would necessitate teams having a known caseload.'

and in *Towards a Healthy Nation*:

'The College recommends that local teams of midwives should be established covering specific-geographical areas ... and should hold their own caseloads.'

It is only sensible to base the bulk of midwifery care in the community. It is after all where the women live, and antenatal care carried out in the home or at a clinic around the corner must be more convenient for a woman than having to go all the way to a large hospital, either on public transport which drops her miles away from the clinic, or in her own car – in which case she finds it impossible to park!

Women have been saying for years and years that it is important to them to have a midwife they know with them during labour rather than a stranger – however kind. At least we are listening!

1978
Micklethwaite, Beard and Shaw
'She would like, if it were possible, to have someone around during her labour who had given her some antenatal care.'

1980
Short Report
'I think this is what women complain about most: they do not have

continuity of care which they want very much during their antenatal visits but certainly during labour and delivery.'
'We recognise the difficulties of providing continuity of care
throughout pregnancy and labour but consider that a measure of it
can be attained by better organisation.'

1981
Kitzinger
'there is an almost complete absence of continuity of care and each
time she attends a woman sees different, anonymous faces.'

1982
MSAC
'Continuity of care. It is important that the woman should be able
to build up a relationship of trust with the staff she meets, and
efforts should be made to involve the same group of staff at each
visit.'

1982
Boyd and Sellers
'I was more relaxed because my midwife was with me.' (p. 145)
'By and large it is the midwife who makes or breaks a happy deliv-
ery.' (p. 123)
'These women enjoyed labour – they were given choice, they were
attended by midwives they liked.' (p. 91)
'My labour was a truly delightful experience ... attended by pro-
fessional people that I regarded as friends.' (p. 87)

1982
RCOG
'It has been suggested to us that women should have the same midwife to attend them in labour as in the antenatal period. We consider this continuity of care to be an ideal aim and it may be
possible in some circumstances.'

1983
Ong, Family Service Units
'Plan effective continuity of care – women should have the oppor-
tunity of building up a relationship with one doctor, one midwife.'

1983
Parents
'Mothers would like antenatal, delivery and postnatal care to be
provided, as far as possible, by the same people. Again and again,

letters expressed the anxiety that arises when seeing a different doctor at each visit to the antenatal clinic, and at being delivered by total strangers – sometimes two different shifts of total strangers if a woman had a long labour.'

1986
Parents
'Good communications between parents and the medical staff were helped where women saw the same people at almost every antenatal visit and were delivered by total strangers. While full of praise for the care they received, many women wished they could have had more continuity of care through pregnancy and beyond.'

1987
Flint and Poulengeris
'I feel that everybody would benefit from knowing the midwife who delivers them. I found this to be extremely important when in labour, I would have been much more nervous and scared if I hadn't known and trusted my midwife.'
'It would be nice if you could see the same midwife all through your pregnancy then during labour.'
'The same midwife should follow the patient from clinic to delivery to postnatal ward and hopefully to her home afterwards.'

THE ORGANIZATION OF TEAM MIDWIFERY

The central concept of working in a small team of midwives is that the women whose care you are providing are enabled to form a close relationship with their midwives. A close relationship is not formed by the woman catching a glimpse of the midwife as she passes her in the antenatal clinic or glimpsing the midwife from the other side of the room at a 'tea party'. Building a close relationship requires a period of discussion and face-to-face chat between the two, preferably on more than one occasion.

If we look further at the model of care suggested by *The Vision* and *The Role and Education of the Future Midwife in the United Kingdom* we can see that most women (about 85%) will be looked after in the community by a small team of midwives who provide the bulk of the women's care. The midwife teams would co-operate with both GPs and consultant obstetricians and the women could see their doctors at specified times during the pregnancy. A *suggested* plan might be:

Midwives at 8, 12, 20, 24, 30, 32, 34, 37, 39, 40 and 41 weeks.
GP at 28 and 38 weeks.
Hospital obstetrician at 16, 36 and 42 weeks of pregnancy.

If the midwives work in a team of five, each woman would be able to meet each midwife at least twice during her pregnancy on this schedule. When the woman goes into labour she can bleep the midwife on call from her team. That midwife can visit her at home to assess her labour progress. The woman will have the satisfaction of having a midwife visit her who she knows. When it is time for the woman to go into hospital the midwife will accompany her along with the woman's husband/partner/mother/friends. The atmosphere that they have already set up at home will continue into the hospital delivery ward. The midwife will continue to care for the woman in labour but if the labour goes on for a very long time into the next 'on call' period, the midwife can stay with the woman or she can call her colleague who is now 'on call' – secure in the knowledge that this woman knows the midwife who is taking over. After the woman has had her baby, she can go home with the midwife and be cared for at home by her team of five midwives – all of whom she knows. If she needs or wants to stay in hospital for a short time, the midwives can visit her twice daily in the ante/postnatal ward.

At the end of this chapter (pp. 210–11) there are two sample rotas which may be useful for you when you set up teams of midwives. They are all based on midwives being on call for 24-hour periods but when the midwife is on call she has a bleep in her pocket *and she is not expected to do any other work* so that she can be free to go shopping, go to the library, go out to coffee, go to a class. Being on call is stressful and it is not fair to either the midwife or the women to expect her also to be responsible for fitting in x amount of postnatal visits, an antenatal clinic and a class when she is on call. It may be that she will volunteer to help with these sometimes but the basic idea is that she must feel free of other commitments.

When the midwives in this type of system are actually called, or are actually working, they keep an account of their hours (form on p. 203) so that, if they are working more than the 150 hours every 28 days that midwives are contracted to work, the team leader (who does not appear on the rota) can take over their work for them and 'pay them back' for any extra hours they have worked.

A formula can be worked out so that each health district can provide continuity of care for all the women in their catchment area. The blank chart on p. 200 shows teams of five midwives working from the community but working peripatetically – being able to bring women into hospital to deliver them and being able to carry out postnatal visits in the hospital as well as at home. Each team of five midwives takes responsibility for 250 women a year, working with obstetricians and GPs as necessary (the male (*sic*) figure to their right).

The hospital-based midwifery team is working closely with an obstetrician (the male (*sic*) figure at the head of the team). They work in a team of seven midwives and carry on working with the usual shifts that hospital midwives do at the moment – early shift, late shift and night shift. They are with the 'high risk' women during their antenatal consultations in the hospital, during labour and on the postnatal ward. They also help with the care of women from the community teams who have to stay in hospital and whose midwives visit twice a day.

There is a skeleton team in the labour ward and ante/ postnatal ward and probably a couple of skeleton staff in the antenatal clinic. If women carry their own notes the amount of administration needed is vastly reduced.

After the specimen sheet (p. 200) are sheets filled in with suggested establishments for a health district with 1,500 deliveries a year (p. 201) and for a district which has 4,000 deliveries a year (p. 202).

A blank specimen chart

OF EVERY

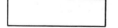

PREGNANT WOMEN

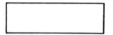

NORMAL PREGNANCIES NEED MIDWIFE CARE

ADVANTAGES

- Continuity of care for women.
- More job satisfaction for midwives.
- Easier recruitment of midwives.
- Quality of care enhanced.
- Domino scheme.
- Midwife to midwife support.
- Liaison with obstetricians and GPs.

HIGH—RISK PREGNANCIES NEED HOSPITAL CARE

ADVANTAGES

- Continuity of care for women who are going through a stressful experience.
- More supportive care for women having problems such as stillborn babies and miscarriages.
- Higher quality of care for women.
- Increased satisfaction for obstetricians working closely with 'their' midwives.

SKELETON STAFF

ADVANTAGES

- A role for part-time staff.
- More streamlined running of wards.

COSTING

ADVANTAGES

- Cheaper than conventional care.
- Quality of care greater.
- Continuity of care for all women.
- No overtime payments.
- Job satisfaction for midwives.
- This health authority leading the way.
- Easier centralisation of maternity services.

COMMUNITY TEAMS

Per 250 mothers
Based in the community providing antenatal care in the community, domino deliveries, and postnatal care in the community.

HOSPITAL TEAMS

Based in hospital providing antenatal, delivery and postnatal care in hospital.

LABOUR WARD

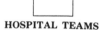

ANTE/POSTNATAL WARD

RESULTS

- Great decrease in hospital stays.
- More women would be in and out.
- Probable decrease in antenatal costs.
- All round cost savings.

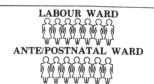

Suggested establishment for a
health district with 1,500 deliveries a year.

OF EVERY

1,500

PREGNANT WOMEN

1,250

NORMAL PREGNANCIES
NEED MIDWIFE CARE

ADVANTAGES
- Continuity of care for women.
- More job satisfaction for midwives.
- Easier recruitment of midwives.
- Quality of care enhanced.
- Domino scheme.
- Midwife to midwife support.
- Liaison with obstetricians and GPs.

5

COMMUNITY TEAMS

Per 250 mothers
Based in the community providing
antenatal care in the community,
domino deliveries, and postnatal
care in the community.

250

HIGH—RISK PREGNANCIES
NEED HOSPITAL CARE

ADVANTAGES
- Continuity of care for women who are going through a stressful experience.
- More supportive care for women having problems such as stillborn babies and miscarriages.
- Higher quality of care for women.
- Increased satisfaction for obstetricians working closely with 'their' midwives.

2

HOSPITAL TEAMS

Based in hospital providing antenatal,
delivery and postnatal care in hospital.

SKELETON STAFF

ADVANTAGES
- A role for part-time staff.
- More streamlined running of wards.

COSTING

ADVANTAGES
- Cheaper than conventional care.
- Quality of care greater.
- Continuity of care for all women.
- No overtime payments.
- Job satisfaction for midwives.
- This health authority leading the way.
- Easier centralisation of maternity services.

LABOUR WARD

ANTE/POSTNATAL WARD

RESULTS
- Great decrease in hospital stays.
- More women would be in and out.
- Probable decrease in antenatal costs.
- All round cost savings.

Suggested establishment for a health district with 4,000 deliveries a year.

OF EVERY

4,000

PREGNANT WOMEN

3,400

NORMAL PREGNANCIES
NEED MIDWIFE CARE

ADVANTAGES

- Continuity of care for women.
- More job satisfaction for midwives.
- Easier recruitment of midwives.
- Quality of care enhanced.
- Domino scheme.
- Midwife to midwife support.
- Liaison with obstetricians and GPs.

14

COMMUNITY TEAMS

Per 250 mothers
Based in the community providing antenatal care in the community, domino deliveries, and postnatal care in the community.

600

HIGH—RISK PREGNANCIES
NEED HOSPITAL CARE

ADVANTAGES

- Continuity of care for women who are going through a stressful experience.
- More supportive care for women having problems such as stillborn babies and miscarriages.
- Higher quality of care for women.
- Increased satisfaction for obstetricians working closely with 'their' midwives.

4

HOSPITAL TEAMS

Based in hospital providing antenatal, delivery and postnatal care in hospital.

SKELETON STAFF

ADVANTAGES

- A role for part-time staff.
- More streamlined running of wards.

COSTING

ADVANTAGES

- Cheaper than conventional care.
- Quality of care greater.
- Continuity of care for all women.
- No overtime payments.
- Job satisfaction for midwives.
- This health authority leading the way.
- Easier centralisation of maternity services.

LABOUR WARD

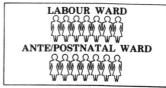

ANTE/POSTNATAL WARD

RESULTS

- Great decrease in hospital stays.
- More women would be in and out.
- Probable decrease in antenatal costs.
- All round cost savings.

Record of hours kept by each team midwife

DATE & DAY	NO. of hours worked	From midnight Saturday to midnight Sunday + ⅔	From midnight Sunday to 6 a.m. Monday + ⅓	From 6 a.m. Monday to 8 p.m. Monday Basic	From 8 p.m. Monday to 6 a.m. Tuesday + ⅓	From 6 a.m. Tuesday to 8 p.m. Tuesday Basic	From 8 p.m. Tuesday to 6 a.m. Wednesday + ⅓	From 6 a.m. Wednesday to 8 p.m. Wednesday Basic	From 8 p.m. Wednesday to 6 a.m. Thursday + ⅓	From 6 a.m. Thursday to 8 p.m. Thursday Basic	From 8 p.m. Thursday to 6 a.m. Friday + ⅓	From 6 a.m. Friday to 8 p.m. Friday Basic	From 8 p.m. Friday to 6 a.m. Saturday + ⅓	From 6 a.m. Saturday to midnight Saturday + ⅓	BANK HOLIDAY (from midnight to midnight) + ⅔					
																No. of hours worked in 28 days =				
																PLUS				
																on extra days—to be carried forward.				
ON CALLS DAY & DATE																				

MONTH & YEAR

MIDWIFE'S NAME

YOUR MIDWIVES

Penny Church is interested in music, sport and reading. She is a dab hand at the guitar. She trained as a nurse at the Westminster and as a midwife at St George's hospital.

Wendy Pearce is interested in music, photography and running. She has a daughter Nancy who is 4, and is divorced.

Claire Neil has 2 children, Marie who is 13 and Vaughan who is 10. She likes music, reading and going to the theatre.

Caroline Flint has 3 children Matthew (18), Rebecca (16) and Tom (14). She likes music, especially Mozart.

Jane Jones paints in water colours—she has had several local exhibitions.

When you have your baby

We want to help make your pregnancy and birth as happy an experience as is possible. During your pregnancy you will be meeting your five midwives: Penny Church, Wendy Pearce, Claire Neal, Caroline Flint, Jane Jones at the !!!!! Health Centre.

They will give you a pregnancy check at:

12 weeks, 20 weeks, 24 weeks, 30 weeks, 32 weeks, 34 weeks, 37 weeks, 39 weeks, 40 weeks and 41 weeks.

You will be seen at the hospital at 16, 36 and 42 weeks of your pregnancy; and you will see your doctor (GP) at 28 and 38 weeks of pregnancy.

When you think that you are

Who's who

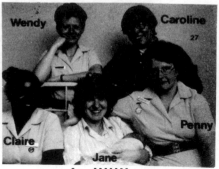

in !!!!!!!
HEALTH AUTHORITY

in labour ring 777 77777, bleep 5555.

Either Penny, Wendy, Claire, Jane or Caroline will phone back. They will either advise you over the phone or come to visit you at home to assess what is happening. When it is time to go into hospital you will go in with your midwife and whoever else you want to take with you.

Your midwife will stay with you until the baby is born. If your labour is very long it will be one of the other midwives you know who will take over.

A couple of hours after the baby is born you will all go home again and your midwives will visit you twice a day for 3 days, and then daily until they feel that you are managing well and that you know how to bath and feed your baby and change its nappy.

If ever you want to contact your midwives for any queries or to talk anything over please phone us on 77777 7777, bleep 555555.

WORKING IN A TEAM OF MIDWIVES

Working in such a team is a new way of working and change always causes pain to those participating in it and those administering it. The team members may feel isolated and confused when starting working in this way – they will need to set up a supportive environment for themselves very early on in their development.

We all need friends and one of the most important aspects of working in a small team of midwives is that the team needs to become its own support group. In order to become a supportive group the team needs to meet at least weekly and the importance of these meetings needs to be recognised – without strength and support from each other any new system will founder. The support must be built into the system and this should be done with weekly meetings.

The weekly meetings need to be a briefing meeting so that all members of the team know what is going on, but, much more important, they need to be an opportunity for all the members of the team to exchange news, views and to really get to know each other. It is important that one person (and that includes the team leader) does not monopolise the meeting. The opportunity to chat is not frivolous – it is this interaction with each other that gives life its meaning, helps us to find out where our place in society is, and adds pleasure to our work. It is not only important, it is crucial.

But to begin at the beginning. Each group has an identity and life of its own, and at the start of each group active measures need to be taken for that group to become cohesive. This needs to be repeated every time a new member joins the group. This may seem a nuisance during a time of frequent changes in personnel but, if special efforts are not taken to form a group each time a new person joins, you will end up with a group which cannot function as a complete unit. The members of the original group will feel close to each other but they will exclude new members of the group; and the new members of the group will feel excluded and inexperienced compared with the original group members and unable to perform to their fullest ability.

GETTING A GROUP GOING

How does a group start? How can we enable it to begin to function as a group? First, by defining for everyone that the object is for everyone to feel part of that group, to belong together, and to feel that this is their space and time. The object of it is for them to feel pleased about meeting each other every week. They also need to know when the meeting is scheduled to end.

Here are some suggestions on how to start group interaction. It can be a good idea to get everyone to move around and to go and shake the hand of each of the other group members, and spend about three minutes introducing themselves. They shake hands again and go on to the next person in the group and do the same, until eventually everyone has introduced themselves to everyone else. Also everyone has touched and been near everyone else so that each member of the group is beginning to get a feel of the other members. When they sit down together they will feel more at ease with each other.

After the first meeting the group can go round the circle and each person says her name and what is uppermost in her mind today, or the worst thing that has happened to her since last week or the best thing that has happened to her since last week. There are many excellent books on forming a group and helping to make it more effective and supportive we have included them in our list of references. It is crucial for the group to form a cohesive and strong *modus vivendi* in order for the group members to function well in their new way of working.

An agenda to which everyone has contributed can also help.

MEETING ON THURSDAY JANUARY 14th
at 4 p.m. in TEAM OFFICE
scheduled to end at 6 p.m.
Car parking (Dora)
Rota swap for April 7th (Caroline)

Rota swap, summer holiday (Libby)
Rota swap – next Monday (June)
Advice on good garage needed (Libby)
Jean French – pre-eclampsia
Mary Greenwich – pre-eclampsia
Shereen Khan – hyperemesis
Things we want to schedule for our next meeting
Any other business

* * * *

You can see from the above list that the needs of the members of the group are rated as highly as the needs of the mothers. You can also see that one of the most pressing needs of the members is to swap parts of the off-duty rota so that their life outside work can be accommodated. One of the ways we can show respect for colleagues is to recognise that they have a life outside work and therefore they need to have their off-duty organised at least a year in advance, but which can be 'swapped' when necessary but only with the consent of the staff member.

There are also touching exercises which encourage good group dynamics. Group hugs can happen when the group forms a circle and hugs itself, or when each member of the group hugs each other member of the group. There are several excellent books on such techniques and these are listed on p. 213. It is important that team members experience their meetings as a sanctuary: laughter will be common and tears will be shed, both these are healing and strengthening and bring people closer together.

Midwives work in an emotional minefield, they are dealing with humans going through the most significant emotional changes that they are ever likely to experience. They have a deep need to have a space where they can share their own feelings. They need friends who understand how they are feeling and who can support them, even if it is only by acknowledging that they have the same feelings themselves. They need to be able to rely on the caring of their colleagues

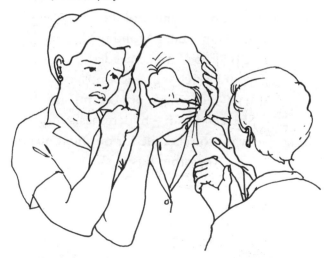

– such a group can be enormously strengthening to its members and can enable them to function at their peak.

In this sort of group midwives are enabled to admit to lacking knowledge on a certain subject. They will dare to say 'I don't understand about *hyperemesis gravidarum*', or 'I've never understood how to judge where the baby's head is in relation to the spines,' and there will invariably be another person in the group who will be able to explain it to her. Often because it is a non-threatening environment, the person who is listening will understand it for the first time. Sometimes a group can decide to explore a topic between them.

Many human anxieties and problems are solved just by someone else acknowledging them. This can only be done in a supportive and private atmosphere. Team members must be able to trust each other (including the team leader) and be sure that what they say will not be around the district tomorrow. This ability to share will come about if frequent meetings take place, at least every week. The team leader must also make sure that she doesn't dominate the group. She must accept that every member of that group is of equal value and importance and that everyone should be enabled to express themselves in the meeting. It is also important that

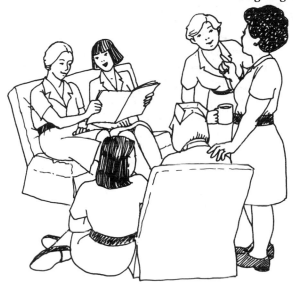

nothing that is said in the privacy of the meetings should *ever* be used against that person.

One of the huge disadvantages of our profession is that we are, as women and as members of a subordinate profession, often as black women, an oppressed group, and the oppressed can turn in upon themselves. But the same socialisation process means that we also have many excellent skills of listening and getting people to talk. Many midwives have, moreover, been on counselling courses and have excellent techniques to help people to tell them their deepest feelings. This ability has to be deeply respected by the person who has acquired it. One of us remembers only too well the assistant director of midwifery services who had been on many counselling courses, who appeared a very sympathetic and warm person. She would urge in an empathetic and caring way, 'Tell me about it,' and within hours of the conversation taking place a garbled and not very flattering version of the story would be told all over the hospital. This type of treatment is extremely destructive of human relationships and should not happen. When midwives are a united team they can bring pressure to bear to stop this sort of behaviour in their unit. On the other hand if that ADMS had herself been a member of a supportive team she probably wouldn't have needed to tell the world what everyone had told her. She would feel strong enough and cherished enough herself to be able to respect another person's privacy.

Throughout this chapter we have mentioned the crucial importance of knowing one's off-duty for months, or even a year, in advance. At present most midwives don't know their off-duty for more than an average of a fortnight in advance. Often, when challenging this, we are told that 'Everyone here knows that they only have to request the off-duty and they will get it', but this really isn't good enough.

Midwives are important and to enable a human being to plan their life, to look ahead with some vision, to achieve the richest and fullest lifestyle, they need to know what they are doing over the next few months and not just the next few days or even the next three weeks.

The ability to plan ahead means that midwives can utilise their time better. Instead of going home after work and slumping exhausted and bored into an armchair in front of the telly, they go home and get ready for the meeting they knew about two months ago, or the concert they booked ten weeks ago. Life is much richer when you can plan ahead. Midwives should be able to enrol in classes which will increase their knowledge – not necessarily their midwifery practice.

On pages 211 and 212 are a selection of off-duties. They are designed for different situations but they may help in your situation. We hope so.

Sample of an off-duty rota for a team of 6 midwives

Midwife	S	M	Tu	W	Th	F	S	S	M	Tu	W	Th	F	S	S
1	L	E	D	E	OC	E	D	D	D	E	E	OC	E	OC	L
2	E	OC	L	E	E	D	D	D	E	OC	L	E	D	E	E
3	D	D	E	OC	L	E	OC	E	OC	L	E	D	E	D	D
4	D	E	OC	L	E	OC	E	OC	E	D	L	E	D	D	D
5	OC	L	D	L	E	D	D	D	L	E	OC	E	OC	E	OC
6	Filling in for annual leave and overtime														

CLASS · MEETING & EVENING ANTENATAL · CLASS · CLASS · MEETING & EVENING ANTENATAL · CLASS

Shows an off-duty rota for a team of six midwives who would be able to provide nearly all antenatal care, all delivery care and nearly all postnatal care to 250–300 women a year.

The sixth midwife is the team leader — she fills in for holidays, study leave etc., and she fills in when a midwife has worked extra hours the preceding month, thus her line is left blank in the sample off-duty, she might also do parentcraft classes and organisational and management activities.

The rota repeats itself every two weeks.

D = Day off.

E = Early shift. On duty at 8 a.m., postnatal care for the women in the postnatal ward who belong to this team, then postnatal care in the community, from 2 p.m. seeing 5–6 women antenatally, off-duty when finished at 4.30–5 p.m. When two midwives are on an early shift they help to relieve the on-call midwife if she needs a break, or if there are two women in labour they look after one of them or they may arrange antenatal classes too.

L = Late shift is from 1 p.m.–9 p.m. in order to see women antenatally in the evening, do postnatal care for women who have delivered very recently and to be on-call for the on-call midwife if she is very overstretched.

OC = On–Call is from 12 midnight until 12 midnight the following day, this midwife is not expected to do anything else than be available for women who bleep her — usually women in labour, but it may be a woman having antenatal or postnatal problems, a crying baby or a heavy bleed for instance.

The times when the midwives have their meeting is marked on each rota and suggestions for classes.

The midwife's name who is doing the antenatal care each day needs to be written in the appointment book so that women are allocated to each midwife and can get to know them all.

Sample of an off-duty rota for a team of 5 midwives

Midwife	S	M	Tu	W	Th	F	S	S	M	Tu	W	Th	F	S	S	M	Tu	W	Th	F	S	S	M	Tu	W	Th	F	S
1	E2	D	E	1-9	E	D	D	D	2	1	E	D	1	E2	1	E	D	2	1	E	D	D	1	2	1	2	2	1
2	D	1	2	1	2	2	1	E2	D	E	1-9	E	D	D	D	2	1	E	D	1	E2	1	E	D	2	1	E	D
3	1	E	D	2	1	E	D	D	1	2	1	2	2	1	E2	D	E	1-9	E	D	D	D	2	1	E	D	1	E2
4	D	2	1	E	D	1	E2	1	E	D	2	1	E	D	D	1	2	1	2	2	1	E2	D	E	1-9	E	D	D
5	Annual leave and refresher course and overtime fill in.																											

An off-duty rota for a team of five midwives who would be able to provide all antenatal care, all delivery care and nearly all postnatal care for 250 women a year.

The fifth midwife is the team leader, she fills in for holidays, study leave etc., and she fills in when a midwife has worked extra hours in the preceding month, thus her line is left blank in the sample off-duty. She might also do parentcraft classes and organisational and management activities.

D = Day off.

E = Early shift. On duty at 8 a.m. postnatal care for the women in the postnatal ward who belong to this team, then postnatal care in the community, from 2 p.m. seeing 6 women antenatally, off-duty when finished (about 4.30–5 p.m.).

1 = First on-call. This midwife is on-call from 8 a.m. until 8 a.m. the next day. She has a bleep and is on-call from home. She responds whenever she is bleeped—usually for women in labour, but also women having antenatal problems when, if it is appropriate, she will refer the E midwife to them, or she will see them herself either at home or in hospital, or postnatal problems when she will respond as with antenatal problems. This midwife goes into the Unit from 4–7 p.m. (or at appropriate times) to perform postnatal nursings on postnatal women who are there from this team, she will also do evening visits for women newly delivered and already at home. (She will negotiate this with the midwife who is second on-call because if she is busy with a labouring woman, or if she is tired, the second on-call midwife will be expected to do the postnatal nursings.)

2 = Second on-call. On-call for the midwife who is first on-call from 8 a.m. until 8 a.m. the next day. Sometimes, this midwife carries a bleep and is on-call from home when for example the first on-call midwife is busy.

E2 = A duty only done at weekends. This midwife comes into the postnatal ward at 8 a.m. and performs postnatal nursings on all the team's women who are there, she then does postnatal care in the community (anyone over ten days is not seen at weekends unless absolutely necessary), she is also second on-call to the midwife who is first on-call until 8 a.m. the following day.

1-9 = 1 p.m. until 9 p.m., only done once a week (a wednesday on this sample off-duty) to run a clinic to see 26 pregnant women (with the midwife on the early shift and the team leader when available).

During the Wednesday clinic all the midwives meet for at least an hour to an hour and a half to discuss their work and to get to know each other well.

Every midwife keeps a record of the time she has worked and is paid back her hours by the team leader who works in her stead. A sample of the chart each midwife keeps is on p.

References

Assocation of Radical Midwives (1986). *The Vision: Proposals for the Future of the Maternity Services*. ARM, 62 Greetby Hill, Ormskirk, Lancs, L39 2DT.

Boyd, C., Sellers, L. (1982). *The British Way of Birth*. London: Pan Books.

Burnard, Philip (1985). *Learning Human Skills: A Guide for Nurses*. London: Heinemann.

Flint, C., Poulengeris, P. (1987). *The Know Your Midwife Report*. London: Heinemann.

HMSO (1980). *Second Report from the Social Services Committee: Session (1979–80) Perinatal and Neonatal Mortality*.

Holloway, Christine and Otto, Shirley (1985). *Getting Organised. A Handbook for Non-Statutory Organisations*.

Houston, Gaie (1984). *The Red Book of Groups and How to Lead Them Better*. London: Rochester Foundation, 8 Rochester Terrace, NW1.

Jelfs, Martin (1982). *Manual for Action*. London: Action Resources Group, c/o 13 Mornington Grove, E3 4NS.

Kennell, J. H., Jerauld, R., Wolfe, H., Chesler, D., Kreger, N. C., McAlpine, W., Steffa, M., Klaus, M. H. (1974). Maternal behaviour one year after early and extended post-partum contact. *Develop. Med. Child Neurol.*, 16: 172–9.

Kitzinger, S. (1981). *Change in Antenatal Care*. Report of a working party set up for the National Childbirth Trust. London: NCT.

Maternity Services Advisory Committee (1982). *Maternity Care in Action. Part 1: Antenatal Care*. Crown copyright.

Micklethwaite, Lady P., Beard, Professor R., Shaw, Kathleen (1978). Expectations of a pregnant woman in relation to her treatment. *British Medical Journal*; 2: 188–91.

Oakley, A. (1980). *Women Confined*. Oxford: Martin Robertson.

Ong, Bie Nio (1983). *Our Motherhood*. London: Family Service Units, 207 Old Marylebone Road, NW1 5QP.

Parents (magazine) (1983) Birth in Britain. A *Parents* special report, 92 (November).

Parents (1980). Birth 9000 mothers speak out. Birth Survey 1986 – results, 128 (November).

Robson, Kay Mordecai (1982). I feel nothing. *Nursing Mirror* (June 23).

Royal College of Midwives (1987). *Report of the Royal College of Midwives on the Role and Education of the Future Midwife in the United Kingdom.* Royal College of Midwives, 15 Mansfield Street, London W1M 0BE.

Royal College of Midwives (1987). *Towards a healthy nation.* Royal College of Midwives, 15 Mansfield Street, London W1M 0BE.

Royal College of Obstetricians and Gynaecologists (1982). *Report of the RCOG Working Party on Antenatal and Intrapartum Care.*

UKCC (1986). *Handbook of Midwives' Rules.* United Kingdom Central Council for Nursing, Midwifery and Health Visiting, 23 Portland Place, London W1N 3AF. Tel: 01 637 7181.

UKCC (1986). *A Midwife's Code of Practice.* United Kingdom Central Council for Nursing, Midwifery and Health Visiting.

Chapter Fourteen

Independent Practice

Working outside the National Health Service and working for yourself has to be one of the most refreshing changes and boosts to any midwife's life. Working in the NHS, however much we applaud its conception, inception and ideals, seems inevitably to smother that which is most creative and free-thinking in individuals. To work independently is to experience great freedom, is to take on much greater responsibility than we are used to, is to experience fear and anxiety, but it is also a time to experience practising truly as a midwife, a time for taking full responsibility for our practice, a time for providing one's own equipment and taking care of it. In other words it is a total life change and a huge and an exciting challenge.

HOW TO START?

If you are fortunate you will be living in an area where independent midwives already work and have set up practices, and you can go along and see them, and ask them to refer any women who they cannot take on – to you. The Independent Midwives Association, 65 Mount Nod Road, Streatham, London SW16 2LP is a source of much support and information for independent midwives. However you do it, it is important to get together with other independent midwives in order to discuss and learn about their special problems and experiences.

Most independent midwives try not to take on more than about two or, at the most, three women a month so that they can give them the fullest care and no anxiety is caused by them not being available when the woman is in labour. Most independent midwives allow themselves a gap of six weeks if they are planning to take a fortnight's holiday.

In some areas, especially if you are well established there

and have been practising as a midwife for some time, it will be easy to establish a practice. In other areas it is more difficult and most independent midwives say that it takes at least a year before your practice is fully established and often two years. If you are working within the NHS you can establish your practice before leaving totally. For instance, if you advertise and take on two women who are due in September and one who is due in November, you can go on working in the Health Service until the end of July or beginning of August and then work on a 'Midwives' Bank' during October. At first your clientele will come in erratically but hopefully, as your practice grows, it will come more smoothly. But midwifery seems always to be either 'feast or famine' so sometimes you will be 'rushed off your feet' and at other times you will have no one due and you feel that the whole idea was a mistake.

The first step to take is to make your service known. It is worth having cards printed. To comply with the UKCC guidelines on advertising, they should not be ostentatious and you should not describe your practice as being superior to any other service.

Home Birth   Antenatal care at home
Mary Bristol
Registered Midwife
Reasonable charges   Tel: 123 4567

---

or

Have you thought about having your baby
at home?

Mary Bristol
Registered Midwife

Reasonable charges

Tel: 123 4567

These cards can be placed in newsagents' windows, sent to your local NCT group, sent to the Society to Support Home Confinements, put in your local paper, local supermarket small ads, sent to your local radio station and sent to the editorial team on your local newspaper. (They might be interested enough to do an article on the services you are providing.)

If you have been unemployed for eight weeks and are receiving unemployment benefit and you can give evidence of having £1,000 you can receive an Enterprise Allowance to help you to set up in business. The best idea is to go to your bank manager and tell him of your plans and to ask him for an overdraft or loan of £1,000. His letter authorising this is then taken to the local DHSS office (address in phone book) and you will be invited to attend an 'awareness day' and given the relevant application form to fill in. An Enterprise Allowance is a guaranteed weekly payment of £40 for a year and, however much you earn, you will still get that weekly cushion to help you to establish yourself.

Having advertised, it is time to start asking around for a good accountant. Many people are worried at the thought of having an accountant, believing falsely that the charges she/ he will make will be more than they can afford. An accountant invariably recoups her fees several times over for you. Having an accountant ensures that you are never worried about your tax position or your National Insurance, as all responsibility concerning this can be handed over to her. Any correspondence concerning your tax can be sent straight to her and you can get on with being a midwife without tax worries. Your accountant will negotiate with the tax office how much you can charge against tax of those expenses 'wholly and necessarily incurred' in the conduct of your profession because, having become self-employed, you will be paying a different type of tax. When you are employed by the NHS or any other employer you will be paying Schedule E tax, which is deducted at source and from which very few allowances can be claimed.

Once you are self-employed you will be paying Schedule D

tax, which means that your clients will pay your directly but you can claim allowances for all those expenses 'wholly and necessarily' incurred in the conduct of your profession. Such expenses are:

- All the equipment you buy for your midwifery practice (stethoscope, sphygmomanometer, thermometers, syringes, bag for holding your delivery equipment, cotton wool, Pinard's, Sonicaid, Entonox, baby scales, measuring jug for blood loss, bedpan, amnihook, bag for antenatal equipment, Syntometrine, etc. etc.)
- Membership fees to professional bodies such as the Royal College of Midwives, Royal Society of Health, Royal Society of Medicine, Association of Radical Midwives, etc.
- Midwives' Information and Resource Service and professional magazines – *Nursing Times*, etc.
- Cost of a bleep.
- Books of a professional nature: this book, other textbooks, books on childbirth, books on being self-employed, books on midwifery, books on obstetric practices.
- Cost of study days, refresher courses, days organised by the NCT or other birth organisations.
- Secretarial help.
- Printing of stationery, cards and case notes.
- Purchase of stationery, pens, exercise books to use as case notes, writing paper, stapler, files, paper clips, stamps, etc.
- Car expenses.
- Telephone expenses.
- Upkeep of your office and where you store your equipment and, if you have them, your consulting rooms.

Most independent midwives, especially at first, do not use consulting rooms; they see their clients in the woman's own home. But however new your practice you will need to keep your notes and documentation in an orderly fashion and not in full view of any visitors who come to your house. You will need a desk, some drawers and/or a filing cabinet, and cupboard space for keeping your equipment in. This is in essence

```
JULY 1987      IN                        OUT      JULY 1987
7.7.87
From Joan Higgs for                 4.7.87
Maternity services    200 —    2 Thermometers, cotton
                                wool, syringes (bill)   10   45
16.7.87                             6.7.87
From Radio Luton                    Metpak for blood
for Broadcast          5 —              tests (bill)   14   00
                                    12.7.87
28.7.87                             Headed note paper   38   50
From Lindsay Steel                      (bill)
for Maternity services  500  00  25.7.87
                                 Book on home
                                     birth (bill)       12   75
```

your office, and if you see women in your own home it will then be your consulting room.

The costs incurred on all these need to be negotiated with your tax office and your accountant will do that. A proportion of all of the above will be used for your work and, obviously, a proportion will be used for your private use. For instance, one sixth of your telephone expenses may be considered as appropriate, or one third, or, if you have a six-roomed house (plus kitchen and bathroom), and you use two of the rooms for your midwifery practice, one third of your house expenses may be claimed against tax. On the other hand it might be a quarter or only one sixth. How will you know how much one sixth of your household expenses are?

The most essential aspect of being self-employed is to get into the habit of keeping up-to-date records of your expenses and your income and *to keep all your receipts*. This is remarkably easy once you have got into the habit. At the start, buy yourself an exercise book, hardbacked for preference, and ruled up as a single entry account book. On the left hand pages write the date and amount of money coming in. On the right hand pages write all the money you spend and clip the

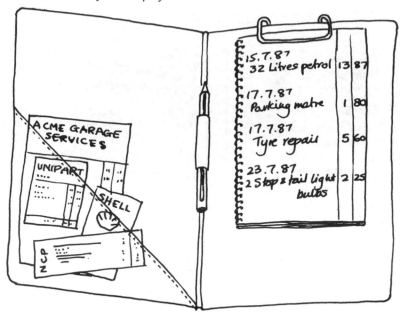

receipts to each page. If you do not have a receipt then quote the cheque number you paid with. When you buy stamps, you can get a receipt or you can buy books of stamps and include the covers of those you use for letters in connection with your practice. With expenses of which only a proportion is claimable against tax, such as household and telephone expenses, it is worth keeping those receipts separately and giving them to your accountant in a bundle (mortgage, rent, rates, electricity, gas, telephone, house decorating, maintenance, water rate, etc.). Car expenses are most easily collected in the car itself.

A clipboard with a pocket and pen holder can be used. Inside this keep an exercise book and write down every time you buy petrol (put the receipt inside the pocket), every time you have to pay for car parking (always ask for a receipt), every time you park in a car park where you stick the car park sticker on your windscreen (keep the sticker and put it in the pocket of your clipboard). If you use a meter obviously you won't have a receipt but write the cost down in your exercise book. Every time you have your car serviced or any repairs carried out on it, keep the bill and write it down in your exercise book. Also the Road Fund Licence, fee for MOT test, car insurance etc.

All this sounds tedious but if you can make it a habit, it is surprising how simple it becomes and how much it becomes second nature.

The next thing to organise is to write to the United Kingdom Central Council for Nursing, Midwifery and Health Visiting, 23 Portland Place, London W1N 3AF, Tel. 01 637 7181, and ask them to send copies of:

Handbook of Midwives' Rules (costs £1 in 1988)
A Midwife's Code of Practice for Midwives Practising in the United Kingdom (free of charge)
Advertising by Registered Nurses, Midwives and Health Visitors (free of charge)
Confidentiality An elaboration of Clause 9 of the second edition of the UKCC's *Code of Professional Conduct for the Nurse, Midwife and Health Visitor* (free of charge)

When your handbooks have arrived, read through them carefully and highlight or underline every sentence which applies to you and your practice. Re-read these sentences weekly so that you will get to know by heart those parts of the Rules and Code of Practice which relate to you. The great strength of our profession is that we have rules, and if you keep within the rules and adhere to the Code of Practice you are safe from blame and accusation. (Chapter Nine deals with the rules very fully.)

Having organised your advertising it is now time to wait for women to contact you and to build up your equipment bit by bit. Here is a list which an independent midwife who has been in practice for a couple of years carries. It starts at the most necessary and goes down to the equipment you could buy when you are more established (or can afford it).

Pinard's stethoscope
Stethoscope
Sphygmomanometer

Urine reagent sticks
Thermometer
Sterilised gloves
Mucus extractors
Sterile cord ligature or sterilised cord clamps
Receiver with lid containing:
    2 pairs of large Spencer Wells artery forceps
    1 pair of scissors
    1 plain dissecting forceps
    1 stitch holder
Syntometrine
Syringes and needles
Ergometrine tablets
Baby resuscitation bag and mask
Entonox
Suture materials
Lignocaine
Intravenous-giving equipment
2 bottles of intravenous Haemaccel
Inco pads
2 catheters
Amnihooks
Amnicators
Tape measure
Baby scales
A large floor covering
Sanitary towels
Cotton wool
Baby oxygen
Neonatal laryngoscope
Red and black pens and scissors
Comfortable clean clothes for the delivery (e.g. T-shirt and loose trousers)

There is a list of stockists at the end of the book. You should always ask for a discount and will often receive a 'professional discount'.

When the first woman telephones you and asks you if you

will come and see her with the idea of booking her, it is a bonus if she is in early pregnancy, but many women only decide at the last minute that they really can't go through with having the baby in hospital. This is a pity because the greatest pleasure is to be gained from getting to know a woman during her pregnancy, labour and postnatally.

Before you advertise for bookings, you will need to have decided how much you are going to charge. Everyone seems to work their charges out in a different way and, as midwives (or is it because we are women?), we find it very difficult to ask for reasonable amounts from people and tend to undervalue ourselves greatly. If this is to be your full-time job you have to make it pay: it needs to cover your rent or mortgage, your car, it needs to clothe you and buy your food, pay for your holidays and hobbies. It might be an idea to work out how much you earn now. If you are working full-time you are working for 225 days a year (this excludes holidays and days off). When working for 7 hours a day, you work a total of 1,575 hours a year. Work out your net salary, divide your net salary by 1,575 and you will see how much you earn per hour at the moment. You probably need to charge at least twice or even three times that amount from your clients, because you also have to pay for all your equipment and you will probably not be employed for a full 1,575 hours at first.

Some independent midwives calculate their fees on £15 or £20 per hour (in 1989). They calculate that the woman receives at least 20 hours of antenatal care, 24 hours of labour care and at least 20 hours of postnatal care and they multiply accordingly. In practice most independent midwives charge what everyone else charges locally, but don't be too influenced by that amount – invariably the midwives in your locality will be undervaluing their services. The psychology of finance is a fascinating and complex subject and it is always easier to quote your maximum price and be able to come down if the woman is having difficulties. It is impossible to increase your charges once you have quoted a price.

Only you can make the final financial decisions although you can get help from your accountant, who will help you to be more balanced about the service you are providing and its worth. Ask how much the private obstetricians are charging for consultations in your area. Are they doing anything very different from you? They may have glamorous consulting rooms – but your women don't have to travel, they sit in their homes and wait for you to visit them. They don't have to wait to be seen – they can get on with their lives until you come – no disturbance for them, and no disturbance for their other children.

It has also to be said that there are many women who just cannot afford fees. If they want to have the service that you are providing them it might be possible to charge them in kind – for every hour of care that you give them, they give you an equal number of hours of knitting/housework/painting help/ironing/cooking/typing/gardening/childcare. Whatever you decide to do it is always easier to make a definite agreement and write it down and for you both to have a copy.

For instance, if you decide that your fees are going to be £1,000 for the whole continuum of midwifery care throughout pregnancy, labour and the puerperium and a woman rings you up and says that she would like to discuss having her baby at home with you, you could describe your services and how much you charge and suggest a consultation so that you can go into it all in more detail and decide whether you are right for each other. Tell her that the consultation will cost £25, which will be deducted from the total amount if she decides to take you on. You go for the consultation visit and, because you have discussed it beforehand, the woman will give you a cheque for your visit. If you hadn't discussed it beforehand, you would be sitting there thinking of how to bring up the question of money and in your head you would be reducing the amount to make it feel easier and you would end up feeling embarrassed and confused and probably with no payment. It is only fair to your client to let her know what you expect of her, then she can be clear and the relationship can be unfettered with thoughts of money, because that has all been dealt with.

SAMPLE PAYMENT SCHEDULE 1

Name . . . .

Total amount agreed . . . .

Amount agreed to be paid at booking . . . .

Amount paid . . . .   Date . . . .

Amount agreed to be paid at 36 weeks . . . .

Amount paid . . . .   Date . . . .

Amount agreed to be paid at delivery . . . .

Amount paid . . . .   Date . . . .

Midwives invariably find it very difficult to ask people for payment – and they consistently undervalue their services. If you find it too difficult to ask on your own account, please remember that when you charge a pittance for your services you are undervaluing our services too. You are saying that all our years of work and experience are worthless – so please don't.

If the woman decides to take you on, you then ask her how she would like to pay – suggesting that some people like to pay £200 a month, others choose to pay £400 at booking, £300 at 36 weeks of pregnancy and £300 after delivery – you then need to type this out with a copy for yourself. Here are some possible payment schedules (pp. 225–227).

With these sort of schedules people will pay you as and when their payments are due and you will usually have no further problems with your fees, and you can get on and concentrate on the relationship you are building up with the parents.

When you have a woman who has booked with you, you will then need to write to the local supervisor of midwives, for example, as illustrated on p. 228.

SAMPLE PAYMENT SCHEDULE 2

Name . . . .

Total amount agreed . . . .

Less first consultation fee . . . .

Actual total . . . .

Amount agreed to be paid in June . . . .

Amount paid . . . .   Date . . . .

Amount agreed to be paid in July . . . .

Amount paid . . . .   Date . . . .

Amount agreed to be paid in August . . . .

Amount paid . . . .   Date . . . .

Amount agreed to be paid in September . . . .

Amount paid . . . .   Date . . . .

Amount agreed to be paid in October . . . .

Amount paid . . . .   Date . . . .

Amount agreed to be paid in November . . . .

Amount paid . . . .   Date . . . .

Amount agreed to be paid in December . . . .

Amount paid . . . .   Date . . . .

SAMPLE PAYMENT SCHEDULE 3

Probable amount of midwifery time given = 60 hours

To be repaid with 60 hours of other work from Joan and Meg

REPAYMENT WORK

2 hours repaid by.............. doing..............

2 hours repaid by.............. doing..............

2 hours repaid by.............. doing..............

2 hours repaid by.............. doing..............

2 hours repaid by.............. doing..............

2 hours repaid by.............. doing..............

2 hours repaid by.............. doing..............

2 hours repaid by.............. doing..............

2 hours repaid by.............. doing..............

2 hours repaid by.............. doing..............

2 hours repaid by.............. doing..............

2 hours repaid by.............. doing..............

2 hours repaid by.............. doing..............

2 hours repaid by.............. doing..............

2 hours repaid by.............. doing..............

Carol Frankham
RGN RM ADM
14 St Oswald Road
Burnton
Wrigtown
AB3 MN7

April 10th 1989

Miss Royanne Philip
Supervisor of Midwives
Buckton Hospital
Fallow Lane
Wrigtown

Dear Miss Philip,

I am writing to ask you to send me a notification of intention to practise please as I have today booked Mrs Janet Baker, 24 Swallow Square, Wrigtown for delivery at home in October with myself acting in an independent capacity.

Nearer the time could you also send me a Birth Notification Form and a Guthrie Test Form.

I have written to Mrs Baker's GP, Dr Floris of 63 Manning Grove to ask her if she is willing to provide medical cover for the delivery. If she is not willing I will inform you and in the case of any deviation from the norm in the health of either mother or baby I will refer the mother or baby to the registrar on call for obstetrics or paediatrics at Buckton Hospital.

Yours sincerely,

Following your letter you will receive a Notification of Intention to Practise form and a written reply which could vary from 'Nice to hear from you, hope all goes well. Let me know if you need any help or support at any time' to a request to go and see the supervisor and to bring your records and equipment for her to see.

If this is the first woman you have booked you won't have anything written in your register (obtainable from Hymns Ancient and Modern, St Mary's Works, St Mary's Plain, Norwich, Norfolk NR3 3BH. Telephone 0603 612 914 to ask for up-to-date price), but you will have notes that you are preparing for this woman. These can be on a form typed, or photocopied, by you. Notes can be very interesting if they are seen as a dialogue between the woman and the midwife and both fill them in. An example of an independent midwife's notes is at the end of this chapter (p. 243). When a woman and her baby are discharged from care, the midwife can photocopy the notes for the couple to keep.

When you go to see the supervisor with your equipment it may be impracticable to carry everything into the hospital, so it is perfectly acceptable to show the supervisor everything you have with you and then to describe all the other things you have, or are going to borrow from another independent midwife. Sometimes the supervisor may feel able to lend you some equipment but usually that is impossible because she is existing on the minimum of equipment herself.

The visit to the supervisor should not be an ordeal but a pleasant experience. She is there to support and guide you in your professional capacity. She is not your employer so she is not able to tell you exactly how to practise, but she is there to ensure that women are safely looked after, and she is there as your guide, counsellor and friend. If she begins to fire questions at you which make you feel nervous just answer 'Yes – I must go away and think about that.' Then when you leave make sure that you do think about any emergencies which could happen at home so that you are prepared for the unusual.

It is essential that the notes are *your* notes. It is inadvisable to use hospital notes if you are offered them. This is because there can be many problems if either the woman has to be transferred into hospital (you then lose your notes into the system) or if there are any queries about the care of the woman (the supervisor can ask you for the notes and you can then lose them because written all over them is ST BEATRIX HOSPITAL, making it difficult for you to say 'These are my notes – please give them back to me.' They are not obviously your notes; they are notes belonging to St Beatrix Hospital).

An example of an independent midwife's notes follows. They record the emotions and events of the woman and the midwife, and the diary of this pregnancy is kept by both of them. It is nice to give the woman a copy of her notes to keep, but the midwife must keep the top copy indefinitely. If she ever has problems in storing them she needs to hand them over to the local supervising authority.

References

UKCC. (1985). *Advertising by Registered Nurses, Midwives and Health Visitors*. The United Kingdom Central Council for Nursing, Midwifery and Health Visiting, 23 Portland Place, London W1N 3AF. Tel: 01 637 7181.

UKCC. (1986). *Administration of Medicines*.

UKCC. (1986). *A Midwife's Code of Practice*.

UKCC. (1986). *Handbook of Midwives' Rules*.

UKCC. (1987). *Confidentiality*.

Chapter Fifteen

The Future

The role of parent is an enormous responsibility and needs great confidence to carry off. How do we prepare a woman to take on this enormous responsibility? How do we ensure that she starts on the road to motherhood confident and strong – feeling powerful and competent?

Let us start at the beginning: let us consider what happens to so many women pregnant for the first time. She thinks she is pregnant so off she goes to see:

1 her pleasant friendly **GP**. He may be working with
2 a **community midwife,** who says she will refer our lady to the local hospital. She attends there quite excited and joyful but a little apprehensive. On arrival there she is met by
3 the **receptionist,** who is very nice and fills in a card with things like her name and address, her GP's name and her NI IS number and other personal details. Then she sits down and waits and waits, until along comes
4 a **lady in a uniform** who is very nice and asks for a specimen of urine and goes off with it. Then along comes
5 **another lady in uniform** who takes her blood pressure and directs her to a little room where
6 **another lady in uniform** asks her a lot more questions about her health and about the pregnancy and gives her a little pile of leaflets to read. Next she is directed to another room where
7 **a person in a white coat** tells her she needs to take some blood to test. She is given a white gown with no tapes and told to strip and put the gown on and sit on a chair and wait until her name is called, and then she goes to another room where there is
8 **a doctor** in a white coat, who prods her tummy and examines her internally (which may be the first time she has ever had a vaginal examination). As by this time she

has a full bladder, it is not very comfortable. She has been afraid to visit the loo in case she missed her name being called. The doctor tells her to come back in a month and that she will have a scan. With the doctor there is

9 **a lady in a nurse's uniform** who smiles and seems nice and asks her if there is anything she wants to know. There were a million things she wanted to know before she came, but her mind is by now a complete blank. She feels totally disorientated, humiliated and violated and responds dumbly by shaking her head. Suddenly tears are not far away and she can't wait to get out of the place, which she does in such a hurry that she finds she has left behind, unread, all the leaflets she has been given.

During the remainder of her antenatal care she attends the clinic, sometimes seeing a familiar face but usually seeing different people each time. She will also meet:

10 **the person who does the ultrasonic scan** and
11 **the dietician**
12 **the social worker**
13 **the lactation sister**

When the great day arrives and her labour starts, off she goes to hospital where she meets another set of strangers, albeit kind and considerate ones. If she is lucky she will have (14) a **midwife** allocated to her in the labour ward for the duration of that midwife's shift, but if the labour takes place across shift times that person will change maybe as often as four times during her labour (15, 16, 17). During *her* labour all sorts of things can be done to her on the instructions of a person whom the woman may not have seen at all during the course of her pregnancy and labour (18) the **consultant obstetrician** whom she is 'under'. He (on this occasion let's assume it is a male) will have quite an influence on her pregnancy and labour because, even though he may never have seen her, he has laid down guidelines for all the staff to follow in the light of his powerful position as a consultant obstetrician.

The guidelines which the obstetrician could have laid down may include policies on:

- artificial rupture of membranes
- sedation and analgesia
- catheterisation
- electronic fetal monitoring – and thus immobilisation
- the frequency of vaginal examinations
- how quickly her labour must go and whether it must be accelerated
- nutrition in labour or lack of it

Her labour is managed by midwives whom the woman has never met before and, in a large hospital, is unlikely to meet again. Having given birth the new mother then goes off to the postnatal ward where ... yes, you're right, she meets yet more strangers, **19, 20, 21, 22, 23, 24, 25, 26,** and then back to the community **27, 28, 29** ...

It has been estimated that the minimum number of midwives alone that a pregnant woman will see during her pregnancy is 30 and then there are the doctors, nursing staff, paramedicals, etc. In this sort of set up what hope is there for parents to develop any self-confidence or feelings of being in control of the situation?

Despite the many changes in the pattern of maternity care in Britain in the last fifty years, we have managed to end up with a service that is organised and controlled by persons far removed from receipt of care and where the needs of the organisation are met in preference to the needs of the individual.

There has been growing awareness that all is not well with the present organisation of the maternity services. In 1982, mothers and fathers were sufficiently angered by what they saw as the routine use of inappropriate obstetric technology that 5,000 of them demonstrated outside the Royal Free Hospital in London. Many midwives are 'dissatisfied with the present conveyor-belt system of midwifery care'. The report, *A Study of the Role and Responsibilities of the Midwife* extensively documents underuse of the midwife's skills, and conflicts resulting from the overlap of her role with that of the doctor. The Maternity Services Advisory Committee was aware of the 'numerous consumer complaints about the so-called impersonal nature of care in hospitals, where maternity services are now concentrated'. They recommend effective use of midwives' skills and state that continuity of care is important to enable the woman to build a relationship with the staff. The Royal College of Obstetricians and Gynaecologists report (1982) that a common complaint is that a pregnant woman may see many different doctors and acknowledge that delivery by the same midwife as seen antenatally is ideal. Midwives and mothers want a safe, sensitive service that sees childbirth as a part of life, not as a disease (Association of Radical Midwives, *The Vision*, p. 1).

The Association of Radical Midwives has proposed a new vision for the maternity services in the next decade. It states that whilst recognising and applauding the strides our profession has made, particularly in the last ten years, the crisis is far from over: 'Many midwives feel frustrated with the present segmented pattern of care and find themselves far from practitioners in their own right.' In order to provide any real improvements in the service the combined efforts of users of the service in alliance with the professionals will be needed.

In this day of severe financial restraints upon health resources it is time for the wholly institutional structure to be re-examined. The Association of Radical Midwives fully supports the ideals of the National Health Service and is committed to the implementation of the 'vision' within the NHS.

The basic principles of the 'vision' are:

- That the relationship between mother and midwife is fundamental to good midwifery care.
- That the mother is the central person in the process of care.
- Informed choice in childbirth for women.
- Full utilisation of midwives' skills.
- Continuity of care for all childbearing women.
- Community-based care.

- Accountability of services to those receiving them.
- Care should do no harm to mother and baby.

(The Vision, p. 2)

All branches of medicine are going out into the community – paediatrics, terminal care, psychiatric services. The branch of the service which seems most suited to take place within the community has to be childbirth – a normal healthy life event happening to normal healthy women, which will have a fundamental and far-reaching effect on the family.

We envisage in ten years' time that 60% of midwives will work from community-based group practices. They will provide antenatal care within the community, and early labour care. They will then go with the woman to hospital or stay with her at home if she is having a home confinement. If the baby is delivered in hospital the midwife will come home with the woman and then the team will give her postnatal care. These midwives will work from a variety of places, depending on local need, and be responsible for the total care of the vast majority of women. (85% of women having a baby in Europe do not have complications, according to the World Health Organisation.)

The remaining 40% of midwives will be organised into teams in hospitals and will provide for those women who present with complications or who develop them during pregnancy.

The aim will be to help all women to take an active role in their pregnancies, births and the postnatal period as a preparation for the active and powerful role they are embarking on as parents.

The 'team' concept is growing in popularity in Great Britain but, sadly, this concept is often rendered meaningless as far as women are concerned. It often means only that the midwives in the postnatal ward try to allocate the same midwives to the same women in the postnatal stay, but as many women only stay in the postnatal ward for two or three days, the fact that the woman has seen the midwife on two days running after having met a plethora of other midwives is irrelevant to her feelings about the totality of her care. The domino scheme was introduced to improve continuity of care by community midwives but, as it is at present implemented, it frequently fails to do this. Also never more than 3% of the childbearing population have ever had a domino delivery.

Care must be established around the woman – she should be the pivot around which care is designed. It is not for her to 'fit in' with what we have designed to meet the wants of the doctors, the institution, the health authority policy, the managers and the midwives. Until we shift the balance of power to the woman our efforts at change will be meaningless.

Deborah Farnsworth, MABC president, when addressing the International Confederation of Midwives in 1986 at the Americas Regional Conference in Vancouver, challenged midwives to 'Maintain services at an optimum level, to strive to keep midwifery in high profile and to support those who are struggling to bring midwifery to its rightful place in health care'.

This is what we all have to do – for women, their partners and their children we must be strong. It is midwives who can ensure that the responsibility for the pregnancy and labour is put into the hands of the parents. We make or break the experience of childbirth for a woman; it is midwives who influence what happens to her and how she feels about herself for years and years to come. The responsibility is enormous – but the rewards are immensely satisfying. If we improve our care so that women are strong and confident and supported by midwives who they have been able to get to know – in their own environment within the loving circle of their families, surely the world must become a better place.

References

Association of Radical Midwives. (1986). *The Vision – Proposals for the Future of the Maternity Services*. ARM, 62 Greetby Hill, Ormskirk, Lancs, L39 2DT.

Maternity Services Advisory Committee. (1982). *Maternity Care in Action. Part 1: Antenatal Care*. Crown Copyright.

Robinson, Sarah, Golden, Josephine, Bradley, Susan. (1983). *A Study of the Role and Responsibility of the Midwife*. London: Nursing Education Research Unit, Department of Nursing Studies, Chelsea College, University of London.

Royal College of Obstetricians and Gynaecologists. (1982). *Report of the RCOG Working Party on Antenatal and Intrapartum Care*. London: Royal College of Obstetrics and Gynaecology, 27 Sussex Place, Regent's Park, NW1 4RG.

Appendix

ADDRESSES OF ORGANISATIONS YOU MAY NEED TO USE

Spaces have been left for local contacts that it is useful to know of before the event.

Active Birth Centre, 55 Dartmouth Park Road, London NW5 1SL. Tel: 01 267 3006.

Association of Radical Midwives, 62 Greetby Hill, Ormskirk, Lancs L39 2DT.

My local contact is _____

Association for Improvements in the Maternity Services, Hon. Subscriptions Secretary, Elizabeth Key, Goose Green Barn, Moss House Lane, Much Hoole, Preston, Lancs PR4 4TD.

Excellent Newsletter. I last renewed my subscription (£6) on _____

Association for Postnatal Illness, Queen Charlotte's Hospital, Goldhawk Road, London W6. Tel: 01 731 4867, or 7 Gowan Avenue, Fulham SW6 6HR.

My local contact is _____

Alcoholics Anonymous, 11 Redcliffe Gardens, London SW10. Tel: 01 352 9779.

Association of Breastfeeding Mothers, 131 Mayow Road, London SE26. Tel: 01 778 4769.

My local contact is _____

Association to Combat Huntington's Chorea, Borough House, 34A Station Road, Hinckley, Leics LE10 1AP. Tel: 0455 615558.

Association for Spina Bifida and Hydrocephalus, 22 Upper Woburn Place, London WC1H 0EP. Tel: 01 388 1382.

My local contact is _____

British Diabetic Association, 10 Queen Anne St, London W1M 0BD. Tel: 01 323 1531.

My local contact is _____

British Epilepsy Association, Crowthorne House, New Wokingham Road, Wokingham, Berks RG11 3AY. Tel: 0344 773122.

British Pregnancy Advisory Service, Austy Manor, Wootton Wawen, Solihull, West Midlands B95 6DX. Tel: 05642 3225.

Brook Advisory Centres, Central Office, 153A East St, London SE17 2SD. Tel: 01 708 1234.

Caesarean Support Network, 11 Duke St, Astley, Lancs M29 7BG. Tel: 0942 878076, or 52 Ullswater Road, Tyldesley, Lancs M29 7AQ. Tel: 0942 873473.

My local contact is _____

Child Poverty Action Group, 4th Floor, 1–5 Bath St, London EC1V 9PY. Tel: 01 253 3406 (2–5.30 p.m. Monday to Friday).

Cleft Lip and Palate Association, 1 Eastwood Gardens, Kenton, Newcastle Upon Tyne NE3 3DQ. Tel: 091 2859396.

My local contact is _____

Compassionate Friends, 6 Denmark Street, Bristol BS1 5DQ. Tel: 0272 292778 for bereaved parents.

Cystic Fibrosis Research Trust, 5 Blyth Road, Bromley, Kent BR1 3RS. Tel: 01 464 7211.

Down's Syndrome Association, 1st Floor, 12–13 Clapham Common South Side, London SW4 7AA. Tel: 01 720 0008.

My local contact is _____

English National Board, Victory House, Tottenham Court Road, London W1P 0HA. Tel: 01 388 3131.

Family Planning Association, 27–35 Mortimer St, London W1N 7RJ. Tel: 01 636 7866.

Foresight, Association for Promotion of Pre-Conceptual Care, Old Vicarage, Church Lane, Witley, Surrey GU8 5PN.

Foundation for the Study of Infant Deaths, 15 Belgrave Square, London SW1X 8PS. Tel: 01 235 1721/0965.

My local contact is _____

Gingerbread, 35 Wellington St, London WC2E 7BN. Tel: 01 240 0953 for single parents.

Haemophilia Society, PO Box 9, 16 Trinity Street, London SE1 1DE. Tel: 01 407 1010.

Health Education Authority, 78 New Oxford St, London WC1A 1AH. Tel: 01 631 0930.

HIPS. Help in Plaster and Splints, 22 Claudius Gardens, Chandlers Ford, Hampshire SO5 2NY. Tel: 042 15 68223. For parents of children with CDH.

La Leche League, BM 3424, London WC1V 6XX. Tel: 01 242 1278.

My local contact is _____

Maternity Alliance, 15 Brittania Street, London WC1X 9JP. Tel: 01 837 1265.

Excellent Newsletter – I last paid my subscription (£5) on _____

MENCAP. Royal Society for Mentally Handicapped Children and Adults, 123 Golden Lane, London EC1Y 0RT. Tel: 01 253 9433.

MIND. National Association for Mental Health, 22 Harley St, London W1N 2ED. Tel: 01 637 0741.

Miscarriage Association, 18 Stoneybrook Close, West Bretton, Wakefield WF4 4TT. Tel: 0924 85515, 11–1.30 p.m. and 6–7.30 p.m.

My local contact is _____

Muscular Dystrophy Group of Great Britain. Nattrass House, 35 Macauley Road, London SW4 0PQ. Tel: 01 720 8055.

The National Association for Deaf-Blind and Rubella Handicapped, 311 Gray's Inn Road, London WC1X 8PT. Tel: 01 278 1000.

National Association for the Welfare of Children in Hospital, Argyle House, 29–31 Euston Road, London NW1 2SD. Tel: 01 833 2041.

The National Childbirth Trust, Alexandra House, Oldham Terrace, Acton, London W3 6NH. Tel: 01 992 8637.

My local contact is _____

The National Children's Bureau, 8 Wakley St, London EC1V 7QE. Tel: 01 278 9111.

National Eczema Society. Tavistock House North, Tavistock Square, London WC1. Tel: 01 388 4097.

National Society for Phenylketonuria and Allied Disorders, Worth Cottage, Lower Scholes, Pickels Hill, Keighley, West Yorkshire BD22 0RR. Tel: 0535 44865.

One Parent Families, 255 Kentish Town Road, London NW5 2LX. Tel: 01 267 1361.

Organisations for Parents Under Stress (OPUS), 106 Godstone Road, Whyteleafe, Surrey CR3 0EB. Tel: 01 645 0469.

Prisoners' Wives and Families Society, 254 Caledonian Road, London N1. Tel: 01 278 3981.

Royal College of Midwives, 15 Mansfield Street, London WM1 0BE. Tel: 01 580 6523.

Sickle Cell Society, Green Lodge, Barretts Green Road, London NW10 7AP. Tel: 01 961 7795/8346.

Society to Support Home Confinements, Lydgate, Wolsingham, County Durham DL13 3HA. Tel: 0388 528044.

Spastics Society, 12 Park Crescent, London W1N 4EQ. Tel: 01 636 5020.

Stillbirth and Neonatal Death Society, 28 Portland Place, London W1N 3DE. Tel: 01 436 5881.

My local contact is _____

Thalassaemia Society, 107 Nightingale Lane, London N8 7QY. Tel: 01 348 0437.

Women's Aid Federation, PO Box 391, Bristol BS99 7WS. Tel: 0272 420611.

Many of these organisations are run on a shoestring, so if you write please enclose a stamped addressed envelope.

SUGGESTED NOTES FOR THE INDEPENDENT MIDWIFE

Name
_____

Address
_____

_____

| Height | Shoe size | Normal weight |

Phone number
_____

Partner's name
_____

Phone number
_____

| DOB | Age | Partner's age |

| LMP | EDD | |

Normal period?

Usual menstrual cycle
_____

Occupation
_____

Partner's occupation
_____

Date of booking
_____

Home facilities
_____

Home helps

_____

Date of home visit
_____

GP

_____

Blood group
_____

Number of previous pregnancies

| Live births | Terminations |

| Stillbirths | Miscarriages |

| Money – amount agreed | amount paid |

Booking
Week 36
Delivery

MY PREGNANCY MONTH BY MONTH

Month   Feelings

MIDWIFE'S ANTENATAL RECORD

Visit	Date	Weeks	Ht of Fundus	Pres & Pos	FH	B/P	Oed	Urine	Wt	Hb
1										

Visit	Date	Weeks	Ht Fundus	Pres & Pos	FH	B/P	Oed	Urine	Wt	Hb
2										

Visit	Date	Weeks	Ht of Fundus	Pres & Pos	FH	B/P	Oed	Urine	Wt	Hb
3										

Visit	Date	Weeks	Ht of Fundus	Pres & Pos	FH	B/P	Oed	Urine	Wt	Hb
4										

Visit	Date	Weeks	Ht of Fundus	Pres & Pos	FH	B/P	Oed	Urine	Wt	Hb
5										

Visit	Date	Weeks	Ht of Fundus	Pres & Pos	FH	B/P	Oed	Urine	Wt	Hb
6										

... etc.

FAMILY HISTORY

Inherited disorders

All the methods of contraception you have used

Please fill in

Method	Dates	Suitability for you

Feelings about this pregnancy, e.g. was it planned, if unplanned why did you decide to continue with this pregnancy. Hopes, fears, feelings towards this baby and your present child/children.

Why do you want to have this baby at home?

Partner's reply to question

What do you see as the duties/responsibilities of your midwife?

Partner

Do you exercise? Please specify

Do you plan to breastfeed?

Any thought on how long?

Have you had any opposition to your decision to give birth at home? Please describe.

There are some things which can go wrong without warning during labour and birth and afterwards. If you are low risk the chances of unpredictable complications are low, but there are risks associated with childbirth whether you decide to take on the risks associated with birth in hospital or whether you decide to take on the risks associated with birth at home. You need to think through the risks associated with birth and read about them/discuss them with your midwife. Please share your feelings and thoughts on this aspect of birth.

Partner

Do you sleep well?

How much time do you usually sleep at night?

Do you manage to rest during the day?

For how long?

How much alcohol do you drink?

Do you smoke?   How many?

What changes in your life are you anticipating when your baby is born?

Partner

Previous pregnancies

Please describe your birth experiences. Things that were done to you that you did and did not like. Did you go to antenatal classes and if so whose? Did you gain benefits from them? What things do you hope will be different this time? Partner's feelings too please.

People you intend to have at your birth, why you have invited them and what their specific roles will be.

I am not perfect – like any other human being criticism is hard to take, but please tell me of any aspects of my work you are not happy with. Repressing negative feelings is not useful because they will come between us, and a woman and her midwife need to grow close to eath other.

Is there anything else you would like to include?

PLEASE FILL IN YOUR PLAN FOR BIRTH

Previous pregnancies

Medical history

In hospital?

Rh fever
Hypertension
Thromboembolism
Renal Disease
Cystitis
STD
Diabetes
Respiratory Disease
TB
Psychiatric
Jaundice
Epilepsy
Blood Transfusion
Migraine
German measles

Operations
Herpes
Hepatitis
Skin problems
Asthma/Hayfever
Thyroid
Cardiac
Allergies

Current drugs

RTA

Details

Any problems during this pregnancy?

LABOUR

Date and time _____

History on arrival

TPR _____ B/P _____

Urine _____

Abdominal examination _____

_____

_____

_____

Membranes _____

Vaginal examination _____

_____

_____

_____

Times

Onset of labour _____

Midwife summoned _____

Midwife arrived _____

Dr informed _____ visited _____

Dr summoned _____ visited _____

Membranes ruptured _____ spont/artificial _____

Liquor _____

OS fully dilated _____

Baby born _____

Placenta expelled _____

Length of first stage _____

       second stage _____

       third stage _____

       total _____

Blood loss _____

Placenta

Membranes

Cord

Perineum _____

Observations after delivery   Baby

Temp _____   Weight _____

Pulse _____   Sex _____

B/P _____   Temp _____

Uterus _____   H.C. _____

Urine _____   Length _____

                                Urine or Mec _____

MIDWIFE'S LABOUR RECORD

Date	Time	Pulse	FHR	Contr	B/P	Urine

Date	Time	Pulse	FHR	Contr	B/P	Urine

Date	Time	Pulse	FHR	Contr	B/P	Urine

... etc.

HOW MY LABOUR WAS – FOR ME

This space can be used by the mother to explore her feelings.

HOW LABOUR WAS – FOR THE FATHER

THE FIRST FEW DAYS – A DIARY

To be filled in by both the mother and her midwife.

Index